Certified Professional Coder (CPC®) Exam Study Guide 2023 Edition

ISBN: 9798372646933

DEDICATION

To the hard working students preparing for the medical coding certification exam. Your work ethic and dedication to the medical coding industry will ensure its health and competency for years to come!

Copyright Medical Coding Pro
Published by: IPC Marketing LLC
PO Box 3824
Youngstown, Ohio 44513

DISCLAIMER AND/OR LEGAL NOTICES:

The information presented herein represents the view of the author as of the date of publication. The book is for informational purposes only.

While every attempt has been made to verify the information provided in this book, neither the author nor his affiliates/partners assume any responsibility for errors, inaccuracies or omissions or for any damages related to use or misuse of the information provided in the book.

Any slights of people or organizations are unintentional. If advice concerning medical or related matters is needed, the services of a fully qualified professional should be sought. Any reference to any person or business whether living or dead is purely coincidental.

Quick Start Guide

Start by reviewing everything included inside the study guide. Contents include the following:

1) CPC Exam Overview
2) Quick Tips
3) Mock Exam #1 - 100 Questions, Answers, and Rationale
4) Mock Exam #2 - 100 Questions, Answers, and Rationale
5) Mock Exam #3 - 100 Questions, Answers, and Rationale
6) Over 180 Coding Tips By Category
7) Secrets To Reducing Exam Stress
8) Common Anatomical Terminology
9) Medical Terminology Prefixes, Roots, and Suffixes
10) Notes
11) Scoring Sheets
12 Resources

These resources used properly will give you a good base to prepare for the certification exam.

If you have any questions please email us at support@medicalcodingpro.com.

Best regards,

Medical Coding Pro

CPC Exam Overview

Certified Professional Coder (CPC®)

The CPC® Exam

- 100 multiple-choice questions (proctored)
- 4 hours taken in its entirety in person or online
- One attempt for $349 or two attempts for $449
- Reliable internet connection and external webcam to show face, hands, keyboard and area around the keyboard (about 10 inches)
- Open code book (manuals)

The CPC examination consists of questions regarding the correct application of CPT®, HCPCS Level II procedure and supply codes and ICD-10-CM diagnosis codes used for coding and billing professional medical services to insurance companies. Examinees must also demonstrate knowledge on proper modifier use, coding guidelines and regulatory rules.

The CPC exam thoroughly covers: 10,000 Series CPT, 20,000 Series CPT, 30,000 Series CPT, 40,000 Series CPT, 50,000 Series CPT, 60,000 Series CPT, Evaluation and Management, Anesthesia, Radiology, Laboratory and Pathology, Medicine, Medical Terminology, Anatomy, ICD-10-CM/ Diagnosis, HCPCS Level II, Coding Guidelines, Compliance and Regulatory, (New) Cases. Ten cases will test your ability to accurately code medical record documentation using CPT®, ICD-10-CM, and HCPCS Level II.

Quick Tips (A lot more tips after the practice exams)

1) Code injections with an administration charge.

2) Supervision and Interpretation components require physician supervision. In radiology procedures this means the radiologist has participated.

3) Know the difference between modifier 26 and modifier TC from your HCPCS II book.

4) Diabetes mellitus – etiology code first then the manifestation code.

5) Trauma accident- always code the most severe injury first

6) Tab all your books including CPT, HCPCS Level II, ICD-10-CM, for quick reference.

7) Code burns on the depth of the burn (1st, 2nd, or 3rd degree). Burns are classified to the extent of the body surface involved. When coding burns of multiple sites, assign separate codes for each burn site. Also burns of the same local site (three-character category level, T20-T28), but of different degrees should be coded to the highest degree documented.

8) Multiple fractures, code by site and sequence by severity.

9) If the same bone is fractured or dislocated, code the fracture only.

10) If the question doesn't state open or closed fracture, code as a closed fracture.

11) Late effects (now called "sequela); is a residual of previous illness or injury. Code the residual and then the cause. Reference "late" in the index.

12) Sequence symptoms first if no diagnosis.

13) Study Medicare A, B, C, D

14) Understand modifier 62 co-surgeons (look on exam for surgeon A and B)

15) ***<u>KEEP MOVING, KEEP MOVING, AND KEEP MOVING!</u>***

Mock Practice Exam Questions & Answers

The following is a Medical Coding Pro Mock Exam. You may not use any outside materials for this exam other than the manuals referenced by the American Academy of Professional Coders (AAPC).

To pass the certification exam you must manage your time carefully. If after going through these practice exams you determine that time management is a skill you may need additional assistance with, FasterCoder.com (www.FasterCoder.com) is an excellent tool to help you with this.

Mock Exam #1 - 100 Questions

1. A new patient presents to the urgent care center with a laceration to the left elbow that happened 10 days ago and was not treated. An infected gaping wound was found, with resulting cellulitis to the forearm and upper left arm. Extensive irrigation and debridement using sterile water were performed but closure was not attempted pending resolution of the infection. Culture of the wound revealed streptococcus. The patient received 1,200,000 units of Bicillin CR IM and is to return in 3 days to follow up. The history and physical examination were problem focused.

a. S51.012A, L03.114, B95.5, 99202, 96372, J0561 X 12
b. L03.114, B95.5, 96372-LT, J0561 X12
c. S41.009A, B95.5, 99202
d. S51.012A, 99281, 96372, J0561X12

2. 12-year-old female was chasing her friend when she fell through a sliding glass door sustaining three lacerations. Left knee 5.5 cm laceration, involving deep subcutaneous tissue and fascia, was repaired with layered closure using 1% lidocaine anesthetic. Right knee: 7.2 cm laceration was repaired under local anesthetic with a single-layer closure. Right hand: 2.5 cm laceration of the dermis was repaired with simple closure using Dermabond© tissue adhesive.

ASSESSMENT: Wounds of both knees and left hand requiring suture repair.

PLAN: Follow-up in 10 days for suture removal. Call office if any questions or complications. What are the correct ICD-10-CM and CPT procedure codes? Do not code anesthesia administration.

a. S81.012A, S81.011A, S61.411A, W01.110A, Y92.009, 12005
b. S81.012A, S81.011A, S61.411A, 12002-RT, 12032-51-LT, 17999-51-LT
c. S71.009A, 12032, 12002-LT, A4364
d. S81.012A, S81.011A, S61.411A, W01.110A, Y92.099, 12032-LT, 12004-51-RT

3. Excision lesion on left shoulder, 2.5 x 1.0 x .5 cm, including circumferential margins. Excision lesion, skin of right cheek, 1.0 x 1.0 x .5 cm, including margins. Pathology report states that the skin lesion on the left shoulder is a lipoma and the lesion on the right cheek is a squamous cell carcinoma. The physician progress note states that the left shoulder was sutured with a layered closure, and the cheek was repaired with a simple repair. What are the correct code sets?

a. C44.329, D17.22, 11641-RT, 11403-51-LT, 12031-51-LT
b. C44.329, D17.22, 11641-RT, 12031-51-LT
c. C44.329, D17.21, 11641-RT, 12031-51-LT
d. C44.329, 11643-RT, 12031-51-LT

4. OPERATIVE REPORT

POSTOPERATIVE DIAGNOSIS: Full thickness burn wound to anterior left lower leg. Operation: Split- thickness graft, approximately 35 centimeters; preparation of the wound. Procedure: Left lower leg was prepped and draped in the usual sterile fashion. The ulcer, which measured approximately 8 x 4 to 4.5 cm, was debrided sharply with Goulian knife until healthy bleeding was seen. The bleeding was controlled with epinephrine-soaked lap pads. Split-thickness skin graft was harvested from the left lateral buttock area approximately 4.5 to 5 cm x 8 cm at the depth of 14/1000 of an inch. The graft was meshed to 1 to 1.5 fashion and placed over the prepared wound, stabilized with staples and then Xeroform dressings and dry dressings, wrapped with Kerlix and finally immobilized in a posterior splint. The donor site was covered with Xeroform and dry dressings.

What are the correct procedure codes reported by the physician for this procedure performed in the hospital outpatient surgical suite?

a. 15220-LT, 15221-51-LT, 15002-51-LT
b. 15100-LT
c. 14021-LT, 15002-51-LT
d. 15100-LT, 15002-51-LT

5. OUTPATIENT REPORT

POSTOPERATIVE DIAGNOSIS: Basal Cell Carcinoma of the forehead.
PROCEDURE: Excision of basal cell carcinoma with split-thickness skin graft.

The patient was given a local IV sedation and taken to the operating room suite. The face and right thigh were prepped with pHisoHex soap. The cancer was outlined for excision. The cancer measured approximately 2.5 cm in diameter. The forehead was in filtrated with 1% Xylocaine with 1:1,000,000 epinephrine. The cancer was excised and carried down to the frontalis muscle. The area of the excision measured 5 x 4 cm in total. A suture was placed at the 12 o'clock position. The specimen was sent to pathology for frozen section.

Attention was then turned to the skin graft. A pattern of the defect was transferred to the left anterior thigh using a new needle. A local infiltration was performed on the thigh. Using a free-hand knife, a split-thickness skin graft was harvested. The thigh was treated with Tegaderm and a wrap around kerlix and ace wrap. The skin graft was applied and sutured to the forehead defect with running 5-0 plain catgut.

Xeroform with cotton soaked in glycerin was sutured with 4-0 silk. A sterile dressing was applied. The patient tolerated the procedure well with no complication or blood loss.

a. C76.0, 15120
b. C44.319, 15120
c. C44.319, 15120, 11646
d. C76.0, 15002, 15120

6. A skilled nursing home patient with an indwelling Foley catheter is diagnosed with a serious urinary tract infection due to E. coli caused by the catheter. The catheter is removed, and a urine culture and sensitivity is performed. A temporary catheter is placed through the urethra, and aggressive antibiotic therapy is begun in the emergency room of the hospital. Which of the following code sets will be reported by the ER physician? No medical evaluation was performed because the patient was evaluated by her primary care physician via telephone with the nursing home staff, and orders were called into the hospital.

a. N39.0, B96.20, 51701
b. T83.511A, Y84.6, 51703, 99281
c. T83.511A, N39.0, B96.20, Y84.6, 51702
d. N39.0, T83.511A, Y83.8, 51020

7. A five-year-old boy was brought to the ER by a social worker who discovered him alone in spasms, and seizures. The Social Worker relates that the child's older sister told her the boy was bitten on the hand by a raccoon he played with 11 days ago. No treatment was sought for the injury at the time, but the area was inflamed and hot. According to the Social Worker, the mother is a drug addict and often leaves the children unattended, illness actually began 2 days ago with a headache and restlessness and inflammation at the wound site. The child expired due to cardiorespiratory failure before any effective treatment could be administered. CPR was preformed but was not successful. The physician's diagnosis was listed as Rhabdovirus from infected raccoon bite, not treated due to child neglect. Critical care was provided for 60 minutes. Which of the following code sets will be provided?

a. A82.9, S61.429A, W55.51XA, Y07.12, T76.92XA, 99291, 92950
b. B97.89, 99285
c. R09.2, R56.9, R50.9, S61.429A, W55.51XA, Y07.12, 92950
d. A82.9, R56.9, R50.9, 92950

8. A 49-year-old female sustained injuries to the forehead, 1.5 cm. and a 1 cm. wound to the eyebrow when she hit her steering wheel with her head. The closure was layered. Code the service only.

a. 12001
b. 12011
c. 13131
d. 12051

9. The burn patient had a 20 sq cm Biobrane skin graft the upper right leg and a 30 sq cm Biobrane skin graft of the lower left leg.

a. 15271
b. 15271-RT
c. 15271-RT, 15271-LT, 15272-LT
d. 15271-RT, 15271-LT X 2

10. Stacey a 35-year-old female presents for biopsies of both breasts. The biopsies were done using fine-needle aspiration including ultrasound guidance.

a. 19100-50
b. 19101-50
c. 10005-50
d. 10005, 10006

11. Don a 36-year-old male, fell 4 feet off scaffolding and hit his left heel on the bottom rung of the support, fracturing his calcaneal bone in several locations. The surgeon manipulated the bone pieces back into position and secured the fracture sites with percutaneous fixation.

a. 28456-LT
b. 28415-LT
c. 28405-LT
d. 28406-LT

12. Tracy a 5-year-old female fell down stairs at a daycare. She hit her coccygeal bone and fractured it. The doctor manually manipulated the bone into the proper alignment and told Tracy's mom to have her sit on a rubber ring to alleviate pain.

a. 27200
b. 27202
c. 27510
d. 28445

13. Fred, a 40-year old carpenter at a local college. While working on a window frame from a ladder, the weld on the rung of the metal ladder loosened and he fell backward 8 ft. He landed on his left hip, dislocating it. Under general anesthesia, the Allis maneuver is used to repair the anterior dislocation of the left hip. The pelvis is stabilized and pressure applied to the thigh to reduce the hip and bring it into proper alignment.

a. 27252
b. 27253-LT
c. 27250-LT
d. 27252-LT

14. A 12-year-old female sustained multiple tibial tuberosity fractures of the left knee while playing soccer at her local track meet. The physician extended the left leg and manipulated several fragments back into place. The knee was then aspirated. A long-leg knee brace was then placed on the knee.

a. 27330-LT
b. 27550-LT
c. 27334-LT
d. 27538-LT

15. By manipulation, under general anesthesia a 6-year-old left tarsal's dislocation was reduced. Correct alignment was confirmed by a two-view intraoperative x-rays. A short leg cast was then applied to the left leg. Code only the reduction service.

a. 28545-LT
b. 28545-LT, 29405-LT, 73620
c. 28545-LT, 29405-LT-51
d. 28540-LT, 73620

16. Dr. Devine applied a cranial halo to Gary to stabilize the cervical spine in preparation for x-rays and subsequent surgery. The scalp was sterilized and local anesthesia injected over the pin insertion sites. Posterior and anterior cranial pins are inserted and the halo device attached.

a. 20664
b. 20664, 96372
c. 20661
d. 20661, 96372

17. Charley was playing in the backyard when his sister fired a pellet gun at his left leg and hit him from close range. The pellet penetrated the skin and lodged in the muscle underlying the area. The doctor removed the pellet without complication or incident. Code the procedure only.

a. 10121-LT
b. 20520-LT
c. 20525-LT
d. 10120-LT

18. Steve presents with a deep, old hematoma on his right shoulder. After examination of the shoulder area, the doctor decides that the hematoma needs to be incised and drained.

a. 10160-RT
b. 23030-RT
c. 10140-RT
d. 10060-RT

19. The surgeon performed an arthrodesis, including a laminectomy of the L1 and L2 segments. Approach was posterior with a posterior inter-body technique.

a. 22630, 22632
b. 22633 X 2
c. 22634 X 2
d. 22633, 22634

20. Brandon comes into the orthopedic department today with his father after falling from the top bunk bed, where he and his sister were playing. He is having pain in his left lower leg and is unable to bear weight on it. Brandon is taken to the x-ray department. After the physician talks with the radiologist regarding the diagnosis of sprained ankle, the physician decides to apply a short leg cast, designed for walking, just below Brandon's knee to his toes.

a. 29405-LT, S93.402A, W06.XXXA, Y92.013
b. 29425-LT, S93.402A, W06.XXXA, Y92.013
c. 29515-LT, S93.402A, W19.XXXA, Y92.013
d. 29405-LT, S93.402A, W06.XXXA

21. A child is seen in the office for a superficial laceration of the right knee. The physician repairs the 3.0 cm. laceration with simple suturing.

a. 12002-RT
b. 13120-RT
c. 12031-RT
d. 12007-50

22. A woman presents to the Emergency Department for a deep 3.5 cm wound of the right arm. A routine cleansing and layer closure was required.

a. 12031-RT
b. 12032-RT
c. 10121-RT
d. 10061-RT

23. Sam is treated for multiple wounds of the right forearm, hand and knee. The physician sutured the following: simple repair, 2.5 cm forearm; intermediate repair, 1.5 cm. hand; 2.0 cm. simple repair, right knee.

a. 12041-RT, 12002-RT
b. 12041-RT, 12002-RT-51
c. 11600-RT, 11420-RT
d. 11400-RT, 11420-51-RT

24. A 69-year-old male is admitted for coronary ASHD. A prior cardiac catheterization showed numerous native vessels to be 70% to 100% blocked. The patient was then taken to the operating room. After opening the chest and separating the rib cage, a coronary artery bypass was performed using five venous grafts and four coronary arterial grafts. Code the graft procedure(s) and the diagnosis:

a. 33514, I25.10
b. 33536, 33517-51, I25.9
c. 33533, 33522, I25.810
d. 33536, 33522, I25.10

25. An arterial catheterization is coded how?

a. 36600
b. 36620
c. 36640
d. 36620, 36625

26. A patient is taken to the operating room for a ruptured spleen. A partial splenectomy and repair of a rupture was done.

a. 38101, S36.032A
b. 38101-58, 38115-51, D73.5
c. 38115, D73.5
d. 38120, S36.032A

27. A 50-year-old patient has a PICC line with a port placed for chemotherapy infusion. Fluoroscopic guidance was used to gain access to check placement.

a. 35656, 77001
b. 36568, 76937
c. 36571, 76937
d. 36571, 77001

28. Code for a transcatheter aortic valve replacement with prosthetic valve via left thoracotomy.

a. 33363-LT
b. 33364-LT
c. 33365-LT
d. 33366-LT

29. For revascularization therapy of the femoral/popliteal territory, how many codes should be used for a combination angioplasty, stent and angioplasty?

a. One
b. Three
c. One but use an Add-On Code for any additional vessels
d. None of the answers are correct

30. PREOPERATIVE DIAGNOSIS: Deviated septum

PROCEDURE PERFORMED: Septoplasty; Resection of inferior turbinates
The patient was taken to the operating room and placed under general anesthesia. The fracture of the inferior turbinates was first performed to do the septoplasty. Once this was done, the septoplasty was completed and the turbinates were placed back in their original position. The patient was taken to recovery in satisfactory condition. Code the procedure(s) and the diagnosis:

a. 30520, 30140-51, J34.2
b. 30520, 30130, J34.2
c. 30520, 30130-51, J34.2
d. 30520, 30140-51, S02.2XXA

31. The patient is seen at the clinic for chronic sinusitis. It is determined that an endoscopic sinus surgery is scheduled for the next day. The patient arrives for same-day surgery, and the physician performs an endoscopic total ethmoidectomy with an endoscopic maxillary antrostomy with removal of maxillary tissue. Code the procedure(s) and diagnosis.

a. 31255, 31267-51, J32.9
b. 31200, 31225-51, J32.9
c. 31254, 31256-51, J32.9
d. 31255, 31267-51, J01.90

32. Gary is admitted to same-day surgery for a laparoscopic cholecystectomy.

a. 47562
b. 47600
c. 47562, 47550
d. 47570

33. Code an excision of a ruptured appendix with generalized peritonitis.

a. 49020
b. 49020, 49060-51
c. 44960
d. 44960-22

34. Code an ERCP with sphincterotomy.

a. 43260
b. 43264
c. 43262
d. 43262, 43273

35. When the physician does not specify the method used to remove a lesion during an endoscopy, what is the appropriate procedure?

a. Assign the removal by snare technique code as a default
b. Assign the removal by hot biopsy forceps code
c. Assign the ablation code
d. Query the physician as to the method used

36. Excision of parotid tumor or gland or both. Once the patient was under general anesthesia, successfully, Dr White, assisted by Dr. Green, opened the area in which the parotid gland is located. After inspecting the gland, the decision was made to excise the total gland because of the size of the tumor (5 cm.). With careful dissection and preservation of the facial nerve, the parotid gland was removed. The wound was cleaned and closed, and the patient was brought to recovery in satisfactory condition. Report Dr. Green's service.

a. 11426, D49.89
b. 42420-80, D49.89
c. 42410-80, 97597, C07
d. 42426-62, D11.0

37. This 10-year-old girl presents for a tonsillectomy because of chronic tonsillitis and possible adenoidectomy. On inspection the adenoids were found not to be inflamed. Only the tonsillectomy was done. Code the tonsillectomy only.

a. 42825, J35.01
b. 42820, J35.1
c. 42826, 42835-51, J35.03
d. 42830, 42825-51, J35.1

38. Which code would you use to report a rigid proctosigmoidoscopy with guide wire?

a. 45303
b. 45346
c. 52260
d. 45386

39. A 63-year-old male present to Acute Surgical Care for a sigmoidoscopy. The physician inserts a flexible scope into the patient's rectum and determines the rectum is clear of polyps. The scope is advanced to the sigmoid colon, and a total of three polyps are found. Using the snare technique, the polyps are removed. The remainder of the colon is free of polyps. The flexible scope is withdrawn.

a. 44110, C18.9
b. 44111, C18.7
c. 45388, D12.5
d. 45338, D12.5

40. This woman is in for multiple external hemorrhoids. After inspection of the hemorrhoids, the physician decides to excise all the hemorrhoids.

a. 46250, K64.4
b. 46083, K64.0
c. 46615, K64.8
d. 46255, K64.0

41. OPERATIVE REPORT DIAGNOSIS: Acute renal insufficiency

PROCEDURE: Renal biopsy

The patient was taken to the operating room for percutaneous needle biopsy of the right and left kidneys.

a. 50200-50
b. 49000-50
c. 50555-50
d. 50542-LT, 50542-RT

42. Code a biopsy of the bladder?

a. 52354
b. 52204
c. 52250
d. 52224

43. OPERATIVE REPORT

DIAGNOSIS: Large bladder neck obstruction

PROCEDURE PERFORMED: Cystoscopy and transsurethral resection of the prostate.

The patient is a 76-year-old male with obstructive symptoms and subsequent urinary retention. The patient underwent the usual spinal anesthetic, was put in the dorsolithotomy position, prepped, and draped in the usual fashion. Cystoscopic visualization showed a marked high-riding bladder. Median lobe enlargement was such that it was difficult even to get the cystoscope over. Inside the bladder, marked trabeculation was noted. No stones were present.

The urethra was well lubricated and dilated. The resectoscopic sheath was passed with the aid of an obturator with some difficulty because of the median lobe. TURP of the median lobe was performed, getting several big loops of tissue, which helped to improve visualization. Anterior resection of the roof was carried out from the bladder neck. Bladder-wall resection was taken from the 10 to 8 o'clock position. This eliminated the rest of the median lobe tissue as well. The patient tolerated the procedure well. Code the procedure(s) performed and the diagnosis.

a. 52450, 52001-51, N32.0
b. 52450, 52000, Q64.31
c. 52450, 52001, Q64.31
d. 52450, 52000-59, N32.0

44. Code reconstruction of the penis for straightening of chordee:

a. 54300
b. 54435
c. 54328
d. 54360

45. New born clamp circumcision

a. 54161
b. 54162
c. 54150
d. 54150-52

46. Sam is a 40-year-old male in for a bilateral vasectomy that will include three postoperative semen examinations.

a. 55250 X 3
b. 52648
c. 55250
d. 52402 X 3

47. Patient is seen for Bartholin's gland abscess. The abscess is incised and drained by the physician

a. 56405
b. 53060
c. 50600
d. 56420

48. A 22-year-old female is seen at the clinic today for a colposcopy. The physician will take multiple biopsies of the cervix uteri.

a. 57455
b. 57461
c. 56821
d. 57420

49. Sara is a 36-year-old female diagnosed with an ectopic pregnancy. The patient was taken to the operating room for treatment of a tubal ectopic pregnancy, abdominal approach.

a. 59121
b. 59120
c. 59150
d. 59130

50. Code a cesarean delivery including the postpartum care.

a. 59622
b. 59400
c. 58611, 59430
d. 59515

51. D&C performed for a woman with dysfunctional bleeding.

a. 58100
b. 58120
c. 59160
d. 57505

52. Incision into abscess of scrotal wall to drain pus.

a. 11004
b. 54700
c. 55100
d. 11006

53. OPERATIVE REPORT DIAGNOSIS: Malignant tumor, thyroid

PROCEDURE: Thyroidectomy, total.

The patient was prepped and draped. The neck area was opened. With careful radical dissection of the neck completed, one could visualize the size of the tumor. The decision was made to do a total thyroidectomy. Note: The pathology report later indicated that the tumor was malignant.

a. 60254, C73
b. 60240, C73
c. 60271, C73
d. 60220, C37

54. Report the codes you would use for burr hole(s) to drain an abscess of the brain?

a. 61253
b. 61156
c. 61150
d. 61151

55. In the operating room the doctor repaired an aneurysm of the intracranial artery by balloon catheter.

a. 61710
b. 61697
c. 61698
d. 61700

56. Removal of a foreign body embedded in the eyelid.

a. 67830
b. 67801
c. 67413
d. 67938

57. Karen is a 13-year-old with chronic otitis media. The patient was taken to same-day surgery and placed under general anesthesia. Dr. White performed a bilateral tympanostomy with the insertion of ventilating tubes. The patient tolerated the procedure well.

a. 69421-50, 69433-51, H66.13
b. 69420-50, H66.43
c. 69436-50, H66.93
d. 69436-50, H67.9

58. Lisa, a 14-year-old female, is seen today for removal of bilateral ventilating tubes that Dr. White inserted 1 year ago. General anesthesia is used.

a. 69424
b. 69424-50
c. 69436
d. 69424-50-78

59. Revision mastoidectomy resulting in a radical mastoidectomy.

a. 69502
b. 69511
c. 69602
d. 69603

60. Biopsy of the upper left eyelid:

a. 67810, 69990
b. 67801
c. 67700-E1
d. 67810-E1

61. Strabismus correction involving the lateral rectus muscle.

a. 67314
b. 67311
c. 67318
d. 67312

62. Excisional transverse blepharotomy with one-quarter lid margin rotation graft.

a. 67966
b. 67950
c. 67961
d. 67961, 15576

63. A 90-year-old patient asks for a second opinion when he was recently diagnosed with bilateral senile cataracts. His regular ophthalmologist has recommended implantation of lenses after surgical removal of the cataracts. The patient presents to the clinic stating that he is concerned about the necessity of the procedure. During the detailed history, the patient states that he has had decreasing vision over the last year or two but has always had excellent vision. He cannot recall a trauma to the eye in the past. The physician conducted a detailed visual examination and confirmed the diagnosis of the patient's ophthalmologist. The medical decision-making was of low complexity.

a. 99252
b. 99242
c. 99203
d. 92002

64. The attending physician requests a confirmatory consultation from an interventional radiologist for a second opinion about a 60-year-old male with abnormal areas within the liver. The recommendation for a CT guided biopsy is requested, which the attending has recommended be performed. During the comprehensive history, the patient reported right upper quadrant pain. His liver enzymes were elevated. Previous CT study revealed multiple low attenuation areas within the liver (infection not tumor). The laboratory studies were creatinine, 0.9; hemoglobin, 9.5; PT and PTT, 13.0/31.5 with an INR of 1.2. The comprehensive physical examination showed that the lungs were clear to auscultation and the heart had regular rate and rhythm. The mental status was oriented times three. Temperature, intermittent low-grade fever, up to 101° Fahrenheit, usually occurs at night. The CT-guided biopsy was considered appropriate for this patient. The medical decision making was of high complexity.

a. 99223
b. 99245
c. 99255
d. 99221

65. A cardiology consultation is requested for a 69-year-old inpatient for recent onset of dyspnea on exertion and chest pain. The comprehensive history reveals that the patient cannot walk three blocks without exhibiting retrosternal squeezing sensation with shortness of breath. She relate that she had the first episode 3 months ago, which she attributed to indigestion. Her medical history is negative for stroke, tuberculosis, cancer, or rheumatic fever but includes seborrheic keratosis and benign positional vertigo. She has no known allergies. A comprehensive physical examination reveals pleasant, elderly female in no apparent distress. She has a blood pressure of 150/70 with a heart rate of 76. Weight is 131 pounds, and she is 5 foot 4 inches. Head and neck reveal JBP less than 5 cm. Normal carotid volume and upstroke without bruit. Chest examination shows clear to auscultation with no rales, crackles, crepitations, or wheezing. Cardiovascular examination reveals a normal PMI without RV lift. Normal S1 and S2 with an S3 without murmur are noted. The medical decision making complexity is high based on the various diagnosis options.

a. 99223
b. 99254
c. 99255
d. 99245

66. A new patient presents to the emergency department with an ankle sprain received when he fell while roller-blading. The patient is in apparent pain, and the ankle has begun to swell. He is unable to flex the ankle. The patient reports that he did strike his head on the sidewalk as a result of the fall. The physician completes an expanded problem focused history and examination. The medical decision making complexity is low.

a. 99232
b. 99282
c. 99202
d. 99284

67. A physician provides a service to a new patient in a custodial care center. The patient is a paraplegic who has pneumonia of moderate severity. The physician performed an expanded problem- focused history and examination. The examination focused on the respiratory and cardiovascular systems, based on the patients' current complaint and past history of tachycardia. The medical decision making was of low complexity and the visit time was 40 minutes.

a. 99236
b. 99342
c. 99342
d. 99308

68. A patient had a bronchoscopy with destruction for relief of stenosis by laser therapy. During this procedure photodynamic therapy by endoscopic application of light was used to ablate abnormal tissue via activation of photosensitive drugs. The photodynamic therapy lasted 60 minutes. How would you report this procedure?

a. 31645, 96567
b. 96567 x 2
c. 31643, 96570-51, 96571-51
d. 31641, 96570, 96571 x 2

69. An established patient is admitted to the hospital by his attending physician after a car accident in which the patient hit the steering wheel of the automobile with significant enough force to fold the wheel backward. The patient complains of significant pain in the right shoulder. After a detailed history and physical examination, the physician believed the patient may have sustained a right rotator cuff injury. The medical decision was straightforward in complexity.

a. 99255
b. 99283
c. 99253
d. 99221

70. An established patient is seen in a nursing facility by the physician because the patient, who is a diabetic, has developed a Stage II decubitus ulcer with cellulitis. The physician performs a detailed history and examination. The medical decision making complexity is moderate and time with patient is 45 minutes. The physician revises the patient's medical care plan.

a. 99310
b. 99309
c. 99315
d. 99238

71. The provider performed an internet assessment for ten minutes, visited three other patients for 5 minutes each, then came back and finished the session for another 20 minutes. The provider called the requesting physician and verbally reviewed the call. Code for this service.

a. 99446
b. 99447
c. 99448
d. This is not a reportable service

72. A 60-year-old male presents for a complete physical. There are no new complaints since my previous examination on June 9 of last year. The patient spends 6 hours a week golfing and reports a brisk and active retirement. He does not smoke and has only an occasional glass of wine. He sleeps well but has been having nocturia times three. On physical examination, the patient is a well- developed, well-nourished male. The physician continues and provides a complete examination of the patient lasting 45 minutes.

a. 99396
b. 99386
c. 99403
d. 99450

73. What modifier would be used to code the physical status for a patient who had a mild systemic disease?

a. P1
b. P2
c. P3
d. P5

74. The qualifying circumstances code indicates a 75-year-old male.

a. 99100
b. 99140
c. 99116
d. 99135

75. This type of sedation decreases the level of the patient's alertness but allows the patient to cooperate during the procedure.

a. Topical
b. Local
c. Regional
d. Conscious

76. What publication is the National Unit Values published?

a. BVR by AS
b. RVG by ASA
c. ASA by RVG
d. RVP by ASA

77. To calculate the unit value of services for two procedures performed on the same patient during the same operative session you would do the following to report anesthesia services.

a. Report only the units for the highest unit value procedure
b. Report only the units for the lowest unit value procedure
c. Subtract the procedure with the lowest unit value from the procedure with the highest unit value
d. Add the units of the two procedures together

78. Code anesthesia service provided for an anterior cervical discectomy with decompression of a single interspace of the spinal cord and nerve roots and including osteophytectomy

a. 00620
b. 00640
c. 00630
d. 00600

79. Per CPT guidelines, anesthesia time ends:

a. When the patient leaves the operating room
b. When the anesthesiologist is no longer in personal attendance on the patient
c. When the patient has fulfilled post anesthesia care unit criteria for recovery
d. When the patient leaves the post anesthesia care unit

80. A physical status anesthesia modifier of P4 means that a patient has:

a. Has a mild systemic disease
b. Has a severe systemic disease
c. Has a severe systemic disease that is a constant threat of life
d. Is moribund

81. Qualifying circumstances anesthesia codes are used:

a. In addition to the anesthesia
b. To describe circumstances that impact the character of the anesthesia
c. To describe provision of anesthesia under particularly difficult circumstances
d. All of the above

82. Anesthesia time starts when:

a. When the Anesthesiologist meets the family
b. When the Anesthesiologist begins to administer drugs
c. When the Anesthesiologist prepares the patient for induction - preoperative
d. When the Anesthesiologist comes to work

83. A 60-year-old female comes to the clinic with shortness of breath. The doctor orders a chest x-ray, frontal and lateral.

a. 71046 x 2, R06.2
b. 71047 x 2, R06.89
c. 71048, R06.09
d. 71046, R06.02

84. A patient presents for an MRI of the pelvis with contrast materials.

a. 72125
b. 72198
c. 72196
d. 72159

85. Code an endoscopic catheterization of the biliary ductal system for the professional radiology component only.

a. 74330-TC
b. 74330-26
c. 74328-26
d. 74300-26

86. Marcy is a 29-year-old pregnant female in for a follow-up ultrasound with image documentation of the uterus.

a. 76856
b. 74740
c. 76816
d. 74710

87. Code a complex brachytherapy isodose calculation for a patient with prostate cancer:

a. 77318, C61
b. 77317-22, C62.90
c. 77772, C52
d. 77300, C52

88. This patient received a prescription for a therapeutic radiology for a cancerous neoplasm of the adrenal gland. What code would you use for complex treatment planning?

a. 60520
b. 77307
c. 77401
d. 77263

89. Because of frequent headaches, this 50-year-old female's doctor ordered a CT scan of her head, without contrast materials.

a. 70450
b. 70460
c. 70470
d. 70496

90. A patient presents to the laboratory in the clinic for the following tests: TSH, comprehensive metabolic panel, and an automated hemogram with manual differential WBC count (CBC). How would you code this lab?

a. 84445, 80051, 85025
b. 84443
c. 80050
d. 84443, 80053, 85027, 85007

91. An 81-year-old female patient presented to the laboratory for a lipid panel that includes measurement of total serum cholesterol, lipoprotein (direct measurement, HDL), and triglycerides.

a. 80061
b. 80061-52
c. 82465, 83718, 84478
d. 82465-52, 83718, 84478

92. Thomas has end stage renal failure and comes to the clinic lab today for his monthly urinalysis (qualitative, microscopic only).

a. 81015, N19
b. 81001, N17.9
c. 81015, N18.6
d. 81003, N18.6

93. This 34-year-old female had been suffering from chronic fatigue. Her physician has ordered a TSH test.

a. 80418, R53.81
b. 80438, R53.82
c. 84146, R53.81
d. 84443, R53.82

94. Surgical pathology, gross examination, or microscopic examination is most often required when a sample of an organ, tissue, or body fluid is taken from the body. What code(s) would you use to report biopsy of the colon, hematoma, pancreas, and a tumor of the testis?

a. 88307, 88304, 88309
b. 88305, 88304, 88307
c. 88305, 88302, 88307, 88309
d. 88305, 88304, 88307, 88309

95. This patient presents to the clinic lab for a prothrombin time measurement because of long-term use of Coumadin.

a. 85210, Z79.01
b. 85210, Z79.2
c. 85610, Z79.01
d. 85230, Z79.2

96. The 62-year-old female who suffers from treatment-resistant schizophrenia comes into the lab today to have a quantitative drug assay performed for the anti-psychotic medication clozapine, a regular white blood cell and absolute neutrophil count due to concern with agranulocytosis.

a. 80159
b. 80159, 85048
c. 80159, 85048, 85004
d. 80159, 85025

97. The 67-year-old female suffers from Chronic liver disease and needs a hepatic function panel performed every six months. Tests include total bilirubin (82274), direct bilirubin (82248), total protein (84155), alanin aminotransferases (ALT and SGPT) (84460), aspartate aminotransferases (AST and SGOT) (84450) and what other lab tests?

a. 82040, 84075
b. 80061, 83718
c. 82040, 82247
d. 84295, 84450

98. The patient presented to the laboratory at the clinic for the following blood tests ordered by her physician: albumin (serum), bilirubin (total), and Urea nitrogen (BUN) (quantitative)

a. 82044, 82248, 84520
b. 82040, 82252, 84525
c. 82040, 82247, 84520
d. 82044, 82247, 84540

99. This male is status post kidney transplant and comes into the clinic for a follow up creatinine clearance.

a. 82540, Z94.0
b. 82575, Z94.0
c. 82565, N19
d. 82570, N18.6

100. An elderly man comes in for his flu (split virus, IM) and pneumonia (23-valent, IM) vaccines. Code only the immunization administration and diagnoses for the vaccines.

a. 90658, 90632, Z23, Z23
b. 90471, 90658, 90472, 90732, Z23, Z23
c. 90471 x 2, 90658, 90632, Z23
d. 90471, 90472, Z23, Z23

Mock Exam #1 - Answers and Rationale

1. a. S51.012A, L03.114, cellulitis secondary to superficial injury, always code the additional injury or ulcer code B95.5, always code bacterial agents after the disease manifestation. 99202 minimal E & M visit for a new patient. Injection, IM, 96372, J0561 X 12, always code the drug and administration of the drug times amount of drug used.

2. d. S81.012A, laceration without foreign body, left knee, initial encounter. S81.011A, laceration without foreign body, right knee, initial encounter. S61.411A, key word: laceration; right hand. W01.110A, Y92.099, Code location and instrument, 12032, 12004-51 code location and size adding together the wounds in the same location regardless how many. Remember that simple closure and single layer are considered the same type of closure.

3. a. C44.329, key word: carcinoma, squamous cell. D17.22, Lipomas are benign and coded by site. 11641-RT, malignant lesion removals are coded separately by site. 11403-51-LT, 12031-51-LT skin lesion removal includes simple repair, code intermediate or layered closures. Both codes are required. See surgery guidelines.

4. d. 15100-LT, 15002-51-LT. code both the wound preparation and then any intermediate graft.

5. c. C44.319, Carcinoma, basal cell of skin of other parts of face. 15120, key word split-thickness. 11646 excision of a malignant lesion.

6. c. T83.511A, N39.0, B96.20, always code reason for the encounter and any manifestations. Y84.6, code the cause 51702 Insertion of temporary indwelling catheter simple.

7. a. A82.9, S61.429A, W55.51XA, Y07.12, T76.92XA, code manifestation and cause codes. 99291, key word critical care for 60 minutes. 92950, Key word; CPR. Be sure to read the guidelines and highlight what is included in critical care services.

8. d 12051 Repair intermediate, wound face.

9. c. 15271-RT; 15271-LT, 15272-LT Application of skin substitute graft to trunk, arms, legs, total wound surface area up to 100 sq cm; first 25 sq cm or less wound surface area. 15272 is the ADD-ON code for the left leg. Often with skin grafts, specific types and brands are identified and have to be cross-linked to the CPT definition. Biobrane: For use in clean and non-infected, superficial partial-thickness burns with minimal involvement of the dermis.

10. d. 10005, 10006: These codes were added in 2019. Key term is “fine needle aspiration;”, Use code 1005 for first biopsy and 1006 for second breast. No modifier is needed.

11. d. 28406-LT key words, manipulated, percutaneous fixation, left heel.

12. a. 27200, open manipulation was never mentioned. The default is to code as closed.

13. d. 27252-LT key words: under anesthesia and pressure.

14. d. 27538-LT key words: fracture, tibial, tuberosity.

15. a. 28545-LT key words: under general anesthesia, dislocation, left tarsal.

16. c. 20661 application of halo, including removal: cranial.

17. b. 20520-LT key words: lodged in muscle, without complication.

18. b. 23030-RT key words: deep, hematoma.

19. d. 22633 Arthrodesis, combined posterior or posterolateral technique with posterior interbody technique including laminectomy and/or discectomy sufficient to prepare interspace (other than for decompression), single interspace and segment; lumbar 22634 is the ADD-ON code for each additional interspace and segment. (Note: 22634 states AMA guidelines “Use 22634 in conjunction with 22633”)

20. b. 29425-RT, application of walking cast; S93.402A, sprain left lower leg; W06.xxxA fall from bed, code location as Bedroom of single-family (private) house: Y92.013.

21. a. 12002-RT simple wound of the extremity. Select for size, location and type. This might be considered a trick question because it is in the 20000 section but that will happen on an actual test.

22. b. 12032 key words: right arm and deep. size of wound.

23. b. 12041-RT intermediate repair; 12002-RT simple repair, Report modifier 51 for second procedure.

24. d. 33536, 4 or more coronary arterial grafts, 33522, an add-on code primary procedure first (AMA "Use in conjunction with 33533-33536), I25.10, native vessels were specified.

25. b. 36620, separate procedure code.

26. c. 38115, repair ruptured spleen D73.5, Infarction of spleen includes splenic rupture non-traumatic. There is no mention that it is laparoscopic.

27. d. 36571, 77001, Fluoroscopic guidance is not included in service.

28. d. 33366-LT is the correct code. Transcatheter aortic valve replacement (TAVR/ TAVI) with prosthetic valve; transapical exposure (eg, left thoracotomy).

29. a. One. Per the CPT Guidelines for this section use a single interventional code, 37230, for the femoral/popliteal territory and do not use Add-On codes. Read and highlight all guidelines notes.

30. a. 30520, 30140-51, Septoplasty, per notes below the code, does not include turbinate resection; J34.2, deviated septum.

31. a. 31255, 31267-51, ethmoidectomy excludes antrostomy must report both codes; J32.9, chronic sinusitis unspecified. See notes below the code. (AMA Guidelines: Do not report 31256, 31267 in conjunction with 31295 when performed on the same sinus)

32. a. 47562, Laparoscopy, surgical; cholecystectomy

33. c. 44960 key words, appendix, ruptured, generalized peritonitis.

34. c. 43262, endoscopic retrograde cholangiopancrateography with sphincterotomy/ papillotomy. (AMA Guidelines: 43262 may be reported when sphincterotomy is performed in addition to 43261, 43263, 43264, 43265, 43275, 43278. Do not report 43262 in conjunction with 43274 for stent placement or with 43276 for stent replacement [exchange] in the same location. Do not report 43262 in conjunction with 43260, 43277).

35. d. Query the physician as to the method used is the best answer.

36. b. 42420-80, total removal with perseveration of the facial nerve; use modifier 80 to show that you are coding for the assistant. D49.89, Neoplasm of unspecified nature of other specified sites.

37. a. 42825, tonsillectomy; J35.01, Chronic tonsillitis

38. a. 45303, proctosigmoidoscopy with dilation

39. d. 45338, code to the farthest placement of the scope and include removal of neoplasm if present; D12.5 benign neoplasm of the sigmoid colon

40. a. 46250, complete removal of hemorrhoids; K64.4, external removal without mention of complication.

41. a. 50200-50, key words percutaneous needle.

42. b. 52204, cystourethroscopy with biopsy

43. d. 52450, 52000-59, must use modifier 59 and documentation must support the separate and distinct nature of both codes, to support the cystoscopy (separate procedure) N32.0 Bladder obstruction.

44. a. 54300 for straightening of chordee (e.g., hypospadias).

45. d. 54150-52, See notes below the code; add MODIFIER-52 when performed without dorsal penile or ring block

46. c. 55250, code is listed as unilateral and bilateral

47. d. 56420, Incision and drainage of Bartholin's gland abscess.

48. a. 57455, Colposcopy of the cervix including upper/adjacent vagina; with biopsy(s) of the cervix

49. a. 59121, no mention of salpingectomy and/or oophorectomy.

50. d. 59515, Cesarean delivery only; including postpartum care

51. b. 58120, excludes postpartum hemorrhage

52. c. 55100, key word: drain.

53. a. 60254, key word: total; C73, Malignant neoplasm of thyroid gland.

54. c. 61150, keyword: drain.

55. a. 61710, keywords: balloon catheter.

56. d. 67938, removal of embedded foreign body, eyelid.

57. c. 69436-50, key word: insertion of ventilating tubes, (For bilateral procedure, report 69436 with MODIFIER 50); H66.93, otitis media, unspecified, bilateral.

58. b. 69424-50, report bilateral procedure (MODIFIER-50) when physician performs procedure on both sides at the same operative session.

59. d. 69603, keywords radical mastoidectomy. NOT modified or complete.

60. d. 67810-E1 always code location with modifier. However, in the real world most carriers only accept RT and LT for epilation, not the E1-E4 modifiers.

61. b. 67311, keyword: lateral.

62. c. 67961, keyword: one-forth.

63. c. 99203, Key words: 90-year old means do not report an E & M consultation code to Medicare, report as a new patient. Also, the physician was charged with diagnosing the patient. Do not bill a consult visit when the patient asks for the second opinion. Detailed Hx and Exam and Medical Decision Making of low complexity = 99203.

64. a. 99223, Key words attending physician, high complexity, comprehensive history

65. c. 99255, Key words; inpatient, comprehensive history, Comprehensive physical examination.

66. b. 99282; Key word; expanded problem focused, low complexity medical decision making and emergency department.

67. b. 99325, Key words: new patient, custodial care center, expanded problem focused, and Medical Decision Making, low. Time 40 minutes.

68. d. 31641, 96570, 96571 x 2. You can find this answer by looking in the index of the CPT Professional under Endoscopy, Bronchi, Stenosis.

69. d. 99221, Key words: admitted to hospital after car accident, lets you know that it is an initial visit. Detailed history and straightforward medical decision making.

70. b. 99309, Key words: established, nursing facility, detailed history and exam, Medical Decision Making is moderate in complexity. Time with patient is 45 minutes.

71. d. The break in time is meant as a distraction. They key to the answer is that there is no mention of a written report, which is required for all interprofessional telephone/ Internet assessment E & M codes. Therefore, this is not a reportable service. If the written report was performed it would have been a 99448 code, adding both times.

72. a. 99396, periodic comprehensive preventive medicine reevaluation and management including age and gender appropriate history, examination (age 40-64). Also called an Annual Wellness Exam or Routine Medical Exam.

73. b. P2, a patient with mild systemic disease.

74. a. 99100, patient of extreme age and younger than 1 year and older than 70.

75. d. Conscious Sedation means the patient can respond to commands. Combinations of pharmacological agents administered by one or more routes to produce a minimally depressed level of consciousness and satisfactory analgesia while retaining the ability to independently and continuously maintain an airway and respond to physical stimulation and verbal commands. Examples of regional blocks include spinals, epidurals or peripheral nerve blocks.

76. b. RVG (Relative Value Guide) by ASA (American Society of Anesthesiologists).

77. a. Report only the units for the highest unit value procedure.

78. d. 00600, Anesthesia for procedures on cervical spine and cord; not otherwise specified.

79. b. When the anesthesiologist is no longer in personal attendance on the patient.

80. c. Has a severe systemic disease that is a constant threat of life.

81. d. Always use qualifying circumstance modifiers in addition to the anesthesia service, when circumstances impact the character of the anesthesia, or to describe provisions that that render anesthesia under particularly difficult circumstances.

82. c. When the Anesthesiologist prepares the patient for induction preoperative.

83. d. 71046, radiologic examination, chest, 2 views, frontal and lateral. R06.02, shortness of breath.

84. c. 72196, Magnetic resonance imaging, pelvis; with contract materials(s).

85. c. 74328-26, interpretation of, Endoscopic catheterization of the biliary ductal system, radiological supervision and interpretation.

86. c. 76816, Ultrasound, pregnant uterus, real time with image documentation, follow-up.

87. a. 77318, Brachytherapy isodose plan complex, C61, Malignant neoplasm of the prostate.

88. d. 77263, keyword(s); therapeutic radiology treatment planning, complex.

89. a. 70450, Computed tomography, head or brain; without contrast material.

90. c. 80050, general health panel, includes DBD, comprehensive metabolic profile, CBC automated and appropriate manual differential WBC count TSH.

91. a. 80061, lipid panel includes cholesterol, serum, total lipoprotein, direct measurement, high density cholesterol.

92. c. 81015, Urinalysis, microscopic only, N18.6, end stage renal disease.

93. d. 84443, Thyroid Stimulating Hormone (TSH), R53.82, chronic fatigue syndrome.

94. d. 88305, 88304, 88307, 88309, surgical pathology code location from which biopsy was taken.

95. c. 85610, Prothrombin time Z79.01 encounter for long term (current) use of anticoagulants.

96. b. 80159: [2014 code] Clozapine; therapeutic drug assay for Clozapine. (This is quantitative; for nonquantitative testing see drug testing 80100-80104). In CPT, 85048 is listed as: Blood count; leukocyte (WBC), automated. Unless the coder works in a lab, this question can be very difficult as the information necessary to code it accurately is not in the CPT manual; additional information is needed. Neutrophil granulocytes are the most abundant type of white blood cells in humans and form an essential part of the immune system. Diagnostic labs also list code 85048 as Absolute Neutrophil Count (ANC), Blood. Both Quest diagnostics and Geisinger medical laboratories consider the one code (85048) sufficient to report both the White Blood Cell (WBC) and the absolute neutrophil cell (ANC) count. The CBC, 85025, and adding code 85004 would be unnecessary.

97. a. 82040, Albumin: serum, plasma or whole blood. 84075, phosphatase, alkaline.

98. c. 82040, Albumin: serum, plasma or whole blood, 82247, Bilirubin, total, 84520, Urea nitrogen (BUN): quantitative.

99. b. 82575, Creatinine; clearance, Z94.0, kidney replaced by transplant.

100. d. 90471, 1st administration. 90472, 2nd administration, Z23, need for influenza vaccine, Z23, need for pneumococcal vaccine.

Mock Exam #2 - 100 Questions

101. Code for a tetravalent, preservative free, flu vaccine for a three-year old girl, injected intramuscularly.

a. 90686
b. 90686, 90471
c. 90687, 90460
d. 90688, 90460

102. The established patient is seen for a comprehensive eye exam (not E & M), fundus photography and the application of corneal bandage lenses for Keratoconus. Code for this encounter.

a. 99215, 92250, 92082
b. 92004, 92250, 92072
c. 92014, 92250, 92071
d. 92014, 92250, 92072

103. The patient is a 55-year-old male. This was a follow up for POAG. The patient had IOP of 22 OD and 24 OS, the optometrist added Timolol Maleate to the patient's Xalatan prescription. The OD performed a Comprehensive Eye Exam, which included ExtraOcular Motility (EOM) Confrontation Fields and a Dilated Fundus Exam, No ROS was taken. The provider performed a refraction exam and GDX of the retina of both eyes.

a. 99215, 92132
b. 92004, 92250, 92015
c. 92014, 92134, 92015
d. 92014, 92134

104. This 70-year-old male is taken to the emergency room with severe chest pain. The physician provided an expanded problem-focused history and examination. While the physician is examining the patient, his pressures drop and he goes into cardiac arrest. Cardiopulmonary resuscitation is given to the patient, and his pressure returns to normal; he is transferred to the intensive care unit in critical condition. Code the cardiopulmonary resuscitation and the diagnosis. The medical decision making was of low complexity.

a. 99282, 92950, I46.9
b. 99283, 92970, I46.9
c. 92950, I46.9
d. 92960, I46.9

105. A patient is taken to the OR for insertion of a Swan-Ganz catheter. The physician inserts the catheter for monitoring cardiac output measurements and blood gases.

a. 36013, 93503
b. 36013
c. 93451
d. 93503

106. Dr White orders a sleep study for Dan a 50-year-old male who has been diagnosed with obstructive sleep apnea. The sleep study will be done with C-PAP (continuous positive airway pressure).

a. 95806, R06.81
b. 95907, G47.30
c. 95807, G47.30
d. 95811, G47.33

107. Mary is a 50-year-old female with end-stage renal failure. She receives dialysis Tuesdays, Thursdays, and Saturdays each week. She sees the physician 4 times per month. Code a full month of dialysis for the month of December.

a. 90960 X4, N18.6
b. 90960, N18.6
c. 90960, N19
d. 90961, N19

108. OPERATIVE REPORT

PROCEDURE PERFORMED: Primary stenting of 70% proximal posterior descending artery stenosis.

INDICATIONS: Atherosclerotic heart disease

DESCRIPTION OF PROCEDURE: Stents inserted via percutaneous transcatheter placement. A 2.5 x 13 mm pixel stent was deployed.

COMPLICATIONS: None

RESULTS: Successful primary stenting of 70% proximal posterior descending artery stenosis with no residual stenosis at the end of the procedure.

a. 92920-RC, 92928, I25.10
b. 92920-RC, I25.9
c. 92928-RC, I25.10
d. 92933-RC, I25.10

109. Dr Green is a neuroradiologist who has taken Barry, a 42-year-old male, with a diagnosis of carotid stenosis, to the operating room to perform a thrombo-endarterectomy, unilateral. During the surgery, the patient is monitored by electroencephalogram (EEG). Code the monitoring only.

a. 95957
b. 95816
c. 95819
d. 95955

110. What part of the neuron receives signals?

a. Myelin sheath
b. Dendrites
c. Axon
d. Cell body

111. Which type of atelectasis is the most common?

a. Inflammation
b. Chronic
c. Compression
d. Absorption

112. What condition is symptomatic of an enlargement of the alveoli and loss of elasticity?

a. Asthma
b. Chronic bronchitis
c. Empyema
d. Emphysema

113. A malignant bone tumor is called ___________.

a. Rhabdomyosarcoma
b. Osteosarcoma
c. Multiple myeloma
d. Chondrosarcoma

114. Name a malignant cartilage-based tumor found in middle-aged and older people

a. Rhadbomyosarcoma
b. Osteosarcoma
c. Chondrosarcoma
d. Chondroblastoma

115. What is the condition called when one accumulates dust particles in the lungs?

a. Tuberculosis
b. Pneumoconiosis
c. Pleurisy
d. Chronic obstructive pulmonary disease

116. What is the condition called where pus is in the pleural space and is sometimes a complication of pneumonia?

a. Pneumothorax
b. Empyema
c. Cor pulmonale
d. Atelectasis

117. What is another name for a compound fracture?

a. Open fracture
b. Closed fracture
c. Complete fracture
d. Incomplete facture

118. Which of the following is NOT an ear bone?

a. Styloid
b. Incus
c. Stapes
d. Malleus

119. The term for a growth plate is?

a. Periosteum
b. Metaphysic
c. Epiphyseal
d. Endosteum

120. Which septum divides the upper two chambers of the heart?

a. Myocardium
b. Intraventricular
c. Tricuspid
d. Interatrial

121. What condition has predominant symptoms of rapid, involuntary eye movement?

a. Astigmatism
b. Nystagmus
c. Diplopia
d. Hyperopia

122. Bacterial cystitis is usually caused by?

a. Staphylococci
b. Proteus
c. Pseudomonas
d. E. Coli

123. Which below is located in a depression in the skull at the base of the brain:

a. Thymus
b. Pituitary
c. Pineal
d. Adrenal

124. The patient, a four-year old child, complained of pain from inside her ear. The doctor found a retained glass fragment in the child's ear.

a. H92.09, H74.8x9, Z18.83
b. H92.09, H74.8x9, Z18.81
c. H92.09, H74.43, Z18.81
d. H92.09, H69.80, Z18.81

125. Acute Bacterial endocarditis due to AIDS.

a. B20, I33.0
b. B20, I39
c. B20, I33.9
d. A80.39, I39

126. Asymptomatic, non-sustained, ventricular tachycardia, there are no prolonged pauses, predominant rhythm is atrial fibrillation with well-controlled ventricular rate.

a. I48.92, I42.8
b. I48.91, I42.8
c. I49.01, I42.8
d. I42.8, I48.91

127. A 50-year-old female patient had two separate carbuncles removed from the left axilla. Pathology report indicated staphylococcal infection.

a. L02.432, B95.8
b. L02.92, B95.5
c. L02.92, B95.4
d. L02.432, B95.7

128. A 55-year-old female with spinal stenosis of the cervical disk C4-5 and C5-6 with inter-vertebral disk displacement had a cervical discectomy, corpectomy, allograft from C4 to C6 and placement of arthrodesis (a 34 mm plate from C4 to C6)

a. M50.90
b. M48.02, M50.221, M50.222
c. M48.02, M51.26
d. M50.90, M51.35

129. A 50-year-old male has staphylococcal septicemia with systemic inflammatory response syndrome and respiratory and hepatic failure

a. A41.2, J96.00, K72.00
b. A41.2, J96.00, R65.20
c. J96.00, K72.00, A40.8, R65.20
d. A41.2, R65.20, J96.00, K72.00

130. The patient, a 21-year old female, has acute laryngitis, chronic fatigue syndrome and presents for both the FLU and pneumococcal vaccine.

a. Z22.9, J04.0, R53.83
b. Z23, Z23, J37.0, R53.81
c. Z22.9, Z23, J37.1, R53.81
d. Z23, Z23, J04.0, R53.82

131. A 5-year-old patient is seen by a physician in an outpatient clinic for chronic lymphoid leukemia in remission and Shiga toxin-producing Escherichia coli:

a. C91.11, B96.21
b. C91.Z1, A04.4
c. C92.21, A41.51
d. C91.Z1, B96.20

132. Discharged with Pneumonia, klebsiella pneumoniae, COPD with emphysema, multifocal atrial tachycardia, middle dementia.

a. J15.0, J43.9, I49.8, F06.8
b. J15.20, J43.9, I49.8, F06.8
c. J18.9, J43.9, I49.8, F06.8
d. J18.9, J43.9, I49.8, F07.0

133. A patient with a history of myocardial infarction is admitted for cardiac catheterization. It is also noted the patient has unstable angina, hypertension, and diabetes with hypoglycemia.

a. I20.0, I10, E13.9, D10.9
b. I20.8, I10, E11.69, I25.2
c. I20.0, I10, E11.69, I25.2
d. I20.0, I10, I21.3, E11.69, I25.2

134. Level II HCPCS codes for drugs are administered:

a. Intravenously
b. Intramuscularly
c. Subcutaneously
d. All of the above

135. A male 62-year-old presents for a digital rectal exam and total prostate-specific antigen test (PSA), which code(s) would is used?

a. G0102
b. G0103
c. G0102, G0106
d. G0102, G0103

136. A Medicare patient, 82-year-old female has an energy x-ray absorptiometry (SEXA) bone density study of two sites of the wrists.

a. G0141
b. G0143
c. G0130
d. G0129

137. A 63-year-old male, Medicare recipient receives 30 minutes of individual diabetes outpatient self-management training:

a. G0109
b. G0176
c. 99213
d. G0108

138. A Medicare recipient presents for an influenza and pneumococcal vaccination.

a. G0008
b. G0009
c. G0008, G0009
d. G0010, G0008

139. General guidelines for HCPCS Level II Coding include:

a. Code directly from the index
b. Search for main terms and any applicable sub-terms
c. Note the reference codes as given in the index
d. All of the above

140. A separate procedure is coded per CPT guidelines:

a. Is considered to be an integral part of a larger service
b. Is coded when it is performed as a part of another, larger procedure
c. Is never coded under any circumstances
d. Both A and B are correct

141. The symbol TRIANGLE before a code in the CPT manuals means?

a. The code is exempt from bundling requirements
b. The code has been revised in some way this year
c. The code is exempt from unbundling requirements
d. The code can be used as an add-on code, never reported alone or first

142. Which is true of the CPT code(s):

a. They describe both physician and non-physician services
b. They are numeric
c. Only physicians can report them
d. All of the above are correct

143. CPT has been developed and maintained by the ___________.

a. American Medical Association (AMA)
b. Centers for Medicare & Medicaid Services (CMS)
c. Cooperating Parties
d. World Health Organization (WHO)

144. This group performs the daily operations for CMS.

a. OIG
b. PRO
c. FI (and carriers)
d. WHO

145. When using the ICD-10-CM

a. Always use the index only when coding
b. Check the tabular before assigning a code
c. It is perfectly appropriate to memorize codes
d. B and C are correct

146. ICD-10-CM codes are composed of 3-7 alpha and numeric digit codes, when using them:

a. Code to the greatest detail
b. It is appropriate to code the 3 digit code when the category is further defined
c. Code to the 4th digit when you don't have the information in your notes
d. B and C are correct

147. When Acute and Chronic Conditions are noted:

a. Always code the Chronic Condition first
b. Always code the Acute Condition first
c. Code both and sequence the acute (sub-acute) code first
d. B and C are correct

148. Which is NOT true of Z-Codes

a. Must always be used at primary diagnosis
b. Are used for other reasons for the encounter
c. Describe signs & symptoms
d. Used to classify diseases and injuries

149. What tool is in place that manages multiple third-party payments to ensure that over-payment does not happen?

a. FUD
b. DME
c. COB
d. PRO

150. A PAR provider:

a. Signs an agreement with the Fiscal Intermediary
b. Submits charges directly to CMS
c. Receives 5% less than some other providers
d. Can bill the patient after payment from Medicare

151. This is a patient classification system that expands the CMS DRGs into four distinct subclasses, which are: minor, moderate, major, and extreme. These subclasses address the patient's severity of illness

a. Case Mix Groups (CMGs)
b. Adjusted Clinical Groups (ACGs)
c. Case Mix Index (CMI)
d. All Patient Refined Diagnosis Related Groups (APR-DRGs)

152. These are assigned to every HCPCS/ CPT code under the Medicare hospital outpatient prospective payment system to identify how the service or procedure described by the code would be paid.

a. Geographic practice cost indices
b. Major diagnostic categories
c. Minimum data set
d. Payment status indicator

153. A service provided by a physician whose opinion or advice regarding evaluation and/ or management of a specific problem is requested by another physician is referred to as

a. A referral
b. A consultation
c. Risk factor intervention
d. Concurrent care

154. A patient is admitted to your hospital six weeks post myocardial infarction with severe chest pains. What would be the correct code?

a. I25.89 Chronic MI
b. I23.8 Acute MI
c. I25.2 Old MI
d. I20.8 Angina

155. In ICD-10-CM when an exploratory laparotomy is performed followed by a therapeutic procedure, the coder lists

a. Therapeutic procedure first, exploratory laparotomy second
b. Exploratory laparotomy, therapeutic procedure, closure of wound
c. Therapeutic procedure only
d. Exploratory laparotomy first, therapeutic procedure second

156. A physician excises a 3.1 cm malignant lesion of the scalp which requires full thickness graft from the thigh to the scalp. In CPT, which of the following procedures should be coded?

a. Full thickness skin graft to scalp only
b. Excision of lesion; Full-thickness skin graft to scalp
c. Excision of lesion; Full-thickness skin graft to scalp; Excision of skin from thigh
d. Code 15002 for surgical preparation of recipient site; Full-thickness skin graft to scalp

157. A patient is admitted in alcohol withdrawal suffering from delirium tremens. The patient is a chronic alcoholic and cocaine addict. Which of the following is the principal diagnosis?

a. Alcoholic withdrawal
b. Chronic alcoholism
c. Cocaine dependence
d. Delirium tremens

158. Code I11, Hypertensive Heart Disease would appropriately be used in which situation?

a. Left heart failure with benign hypertension
b. Congestive heart failure; hypertension
c. Hypertensive cardiovascular disease with congestive heart failure
d. Cardiomegaly with hypertension

159. The Level II (national) codes of the HCPCS coding system are maintained by the ______.

a. American Medical Association
b. CPT Editorial Panel
c. Local Fiscal Intermediary
d. Centers for Medicare & Medicaid Services

160. A cancer program is surveyed for approval by the ________________.

a. American Cancer Society
b. Commission on Cancer of the American College of Surgeons
c. State Department of Health
d. Joint Commission on Accreditation of Healthcare Organizations

161. The purpose of the National Correct Coding Initiative is to:

a. Increase fines and penalties for bundling services into comprehensive CPT codes
b. Restrict Medicare reimbursement to hospitals for ancillary services
c. Teach coders how to unbundled codes
d. Promote correct coding methodologies and reduce improper coding

162. Which of the following could influence a facility's case mix?

a. Changes in DRG weights
b. Changes in the services offered by a facility
c. Accuracy of coding
d. All of the above might influence a facility's case mix

163. The patient sees a PAR provider and has a procedure performed after meeting the annual deductible. If the Medicare-approved amount is $200, how much is the patient's out-of-pocket expense?

a. $0
b. $20
c. $40
d. $100

164. Four people were seen in your Emergency Department yesterday. Which one will be coded as a poisoning?

a. Robert - diagnosed with digitalis intoxication.
b. Gary - had an allergic reaction to a dye administered for a pyelogram.
c. David - developed syncope after taking Contac (over the counter) pills with a double scotch.
d. Brian - had an idiosyncratic reaction between two properly administered prescription drugs.

165. Which of the following is vital for determining why the reimbursement from an insurance company is less than that which was expected?

a. CPT codebook
b. The remittance advice
c. Talking to the patient
d. Knowledge of the individual insurance company's policies

166. Review of patient services needed prior to the patient actually receiving these services is called:

a. Retrospective review
b. Concurrent review
c. Prospective review
d. Discharge planning

167. Which of the following procedures can be identified as "destruction" of lesions?

a. Removal of skin tags
b. Shaving of skin lesion
c. Laser removal of condylomata
d. Paring of hyperkeratotic lesion

168. Which of the following is coded as an adverse effect in ICD-10-CM?

a. Tinnitus due to allergic reaction after administration of ear drops
b. Mental retardation due to intracranial abscess
c. Rejection of transplanted kidney
d. Non-functioning pacemaker due to defective soldering

169. A 89 year old male is admitted from a nursing home with confusion, hypotension, temperature of 103.5 and obvious dehydration. Blood cultures were negative, however urine culture was positive for E.coli. Physician documents final diagnosis as septicemia, septic shock, UTI due to E.coli and dehydration. Provide appropriate ICD-10-CM and CPT codes.

a. N39.0, I95.9, B96.21, E86.0
b. A41.9, R65.21, N39.0, B96.21, E86.0
c. N39.0, A41.9, B96.21, E86.0, R65.20
d. A41.9, E86.0, B96.21, R65.20

170. Incomplete abortion complicated by excessive hemorrhage. Dilation and curettage performed. Provide appropriate ICD-10-CM diagnosis and procedure codes.

a. O03.6, 0UDB7ZZ
b. O03.6, D62, 0UDB7ZZ
c. O03.1, 10D17ZZ
d. O03.4, 10D17ZZ

171. ICD-10-CM codes are sequenced for third party payors based on definitions from the _____________.

a. UHDDS
b. Coding Clinic
c. CMS Coding Guidelines
d. Federal Register

172. Security devices which form barriers between routers of a public network and a private network to protect access by unauthorized users are called:

a. Data translators
b. Passwords
c. Data manipulation engines
d. Firewalls

173. A patient was sent to the surgeon's office as requested by the physician because the insurance company requires a second opinion.

a. 99242-32
b. 99243
c. 99253-32
d. 99203-32

174. Patient has bilateral inguinal hernias, the left is indirect and the right is direct. He has repair of both hernias with mesh prosthesis. Provide appropriate ICD-10-CM diagnosis and procedure codes.

a. K40.91, K40.20, 0YUA07Z
b. K40.90, 0YQ50ZZ, 0YQ53ZZ
c. K40.20, 0YUA0JZ
d. K40.20, 0YQ50ZZ, 0YQ60ZZ

175. Patient has tear of the medial meniscus with loose bodies in the medial compartment of the left knee that was repaired by arthroscopic medial meniscectomy, shaving and trimming of meniscal rim, resection of synovium and removal of the loose bodies. Provide the appropriate CPT code(s).

a. 29804
b. 27333-LT, 27331-LT
c. 29800-LT, 29819-LT
d. 29881-LT, 29874-LT

176. What term refers to a collection of information or data that is organized in such a way that its contents can be queried and relationships created?

a. Database
b. Field
c. Record
d. Table

177. In reviewing a medical record for coding purposes, the coder notes that the discharge summary has not yet been transcribed. In its absence, the best place to look for the patient's response to treatment and documentation of any complications which may have developed during this episode of care is in the ___________?

a. Doctors' progress note section
b. Operative report
c. History and physical
d. Doctors' orders

178. Teena had three babies in four years and she considered that more than enough. During her hospitalization for her third delivery, Teena had a sterilization procedure performed. When the record is coded, the code for sterilization, Z30.2 is ________.

a. Not used
b. Used and sequenced as principal diagnosis
c. Used and sequenced as a secondary diagnosis
d. The only code used

179. Lumbar laminectomy (one segment) for decompression of spinal cord. Provide the appropriate CPT code.

a. 63005
b. 62263
c. 63170
d. 63030

180. Chronic otitis media with bilateral myringotomy and tube insertion using local anesthesia. Provide appropriate ICD-10-CM and CPT codes.

a. H66.93, 69420, 69420
b. H66.93, 69433, 69433
c. H65.119, 69799, 69799
d. H65.199, 69799, 69799

181. Live born infant, born in hospital, cleft palate and lip. Provide appropriate ICD-10-CM diagnosis codes.

a. Q37.9, 0CQ03ZZ, 0CQ33ZZ
b. Q37.9
c. Z38.00, Q37.9
d. Z38.00

182. A marked loss of bone density and increase in bone porosity is called _______.

a. Lumbago
b. Osteoarthritis
c. Spondylitis
d. Osteoporosis

183. Which of the following statements is true?

a. A surgical procedure may include one or more surgical operations
b. The terms surgical operation and surgical procedure are synonymous
c. A surgical operation may include one or more surgical procedures
d. The term surgical procedure is an incorrect term and should not be used

184. Patient with carpal tunnel comes in for an open carpal tunnel release. Provide appropriate ICD-10-CM and CPT codes.

a. G56.00, 64999
b. G56.00, 64721
c. G56.00, 64905
d. G56.00, 64892

185. A four-year-old had a repair of an incarcerated inguinal hernia. This is the first time this child has been treated for this condition. Provide the appropriate CPT code.

a. 49553
b. 49496
c. 49521
d. 49501

186. Patient was admitted from the nursing home in acute respiratory failure that was due to congestive heart failure. Chest x-ray also showed pulmonary edema. Patient was intubated and placed on mechanical ventilation and expired the day after admission.

I50.20 Congestive heart failure
I50.1 Left heart failure
J81.0 Acute pulmonary edema
J96.00 Acute respiratory failure
J96.20 Acute and chronic respiratory failure
0BH17EZ Insertion of endotrachial tube
5A1945Z Mechanical ventilation 24 - 96 consecutive hours

a. I50.1, J96.20, J81.0, 5A1945Z, 0BH17EZ
b. I50.1, I50.20, J96.00, J81.0, 5A1945Z, 0BH17EZ
c. J96.00, I50.20, 5A1945Z, 0BH17EZ
d. 150.1, J81.0, 0BH17EZ, 5A1945Z

187. Female with six (6) months of stress incontinence. Laparoscopic urethral suspension was completed. Provide the appropriate ICD-10-CM and CPT codes.

a. R32, 51992
b. N39.3, 51990
c. N39.46, 51840
d. R32, 51845

188. Staging

a. Refers to the monitoring of incidence and trends associated with a disease
b. Is continued medical surveillance of a case
c. Is a system for documenting the extent or spread of cancer
d. Designates the degree of differentiation of cells

189. Which of the following diagnoses or procedures would prevent the Encounter for full-term uncomplicated delivery, O80, from being assigned?

a. Occiput presentation
b. Single live-born
c. Episiotomy
d. Low forceps

190. Phacoemulsification of left cataract with IOL implant and subconjunctival injection. Provide appropriate ICD-10-CM and CPT codes.

a. H26.9, 66940-LT
b. H26.9, 66983, 68200
c. H26.9, 66984-LT
d. H26.9, 66984-LT, 68200-LT

191. Patient has a year history of mitral valve regurgitation and now presents for a mitral valve replacement with bypass. Provide appropriate CPT code.

a. 33430
b. 33427
c. 33425
d. 35231

192. Which of the following is the term describing a woman who has delivered one child?

a. Primipara
b. Primigravida
c. Nulligravida
d. Paragravida

193. LASER and EGD are examples of __________.

a. Pseudonyms
b. Antonyms
c. Eponyms
d. Acronyms

194. What is the correct sequencing of the codes for a patient who is six weeks post mastectomy for carcinoma of the breast and is admitted for chemotherapy?

C50.919 Malignant neoplasm of the breast
Z85.3 Personal history of malignant neoplasm of breast
Z51.11 Encounter for other and unspecified procedures and aftercare, antineoplastic chemotherapy
Z09 Follow-up exam after surgery

a. Z51.11, C50.919
b. Z51.11, Z85.3
c. Z09, Z51.11
d. Z85.3

195. Urethral calculus, transurethral basket removal of calculus. Provide appropriate ICD-10-CM diagnosis and procedure codes.

a. N21.0, 0TC37ZZ, 0T760DZ
b. N21.0, 0TC37ZZ
c. N21.1, 0T7D0DZ
d. N21.1, 0TND0ZZ

196. The physician has documented the final diagnoses as: acute myocardial infarction, COPD, CHF, hypertension, atrial fibrillation and status-post cholecystectomy. The following conditions should be reported using ICD-10-CM diagnostic codes.

a. I21.3, J44.9, I11.0, I48.91, Z90.89
b. I21.3, J44.9, I50.20, I10, I48.91
c. I21.3, J44.9, I50.20, I10, I48.91, Z90.89
d. I21.3, J44.9, I50.20, I11.9, I48.91

197. HPV or human papilloma virus is...

a. Caused by the spirochete Treponema pallidum
b. A vaginal inflammation that is caused by a protozoan parasite
c. Also known as genital warts
d. Characterized by painful urination and an abnormal discharge

198. Total Transcervical thymectomy. Provide appropriate CPT code(s).

a. 60520
b. 60540
c. 60240
d. 60200

199. You have been assigned to code the cases listed below. Which one will you appropriately assign to I11.0, Hypertensive Heart Disease?

Mallory: left heart failure with benign hypertension
Emma: congestive heart failure; hypertension
Taylor: hypertensive cardiovascular disease with congestive heart failure
Trevor: cardiomegaly with hypertension

a. Mallory
b. Emma
c. Taylor
d. Trevor

200. An established patient was seen by physician in her office for DtaP vaccine and Hib. Provide the appropriate CPT code(s).

a. 90723
b. 90717, 90471
c. 90700, 90748, 99211
d. 90471, 90723

Mock Exam #2 - Answers and Rationale

101. b. 90686: Influenza virus vaccine, quadrivalent, split virus, preservative free, when administered to individuals 3 years of age and older, for intramuscular use. Quadrivalent (aka tetravalent) means the vaccine is a mixture of four flu-types. A "split virus" is chemically disrupted using a non-ionic surfactant, which is further purified. Bivalent is two and trivalent is three. Report the vaccine admin codes 90471-74 in addition to codes 90476-90749.

102. d 92014 comprehensive eye exam. 99250 Fundus photography. Note: for keratoconus. 92072 Fitting of contact lens for management of keratoconus, initial fitting.

103. c. Key Hints here: 55-year old is not a Medicare patient, POAG is Primary Angle Glaucoma, IOP is IntraOcular Pressure The Comprehensive Eye exam is a 92014 code and not an E & M code. Clues are the two included tests (EOM and CF) and that no ROS was done (not need for 92xxx codes) GDX HRT and OCT are all diagnostic tests coded as Scanning Computerized Ophthalmic Diagnostic Imaging (SCODI) 9213x, 92134 is the correct code. Code 92015 for the refraction services. Determination of refractive state.

104. c. 92950, Cardiopulmonary resuscitation (eg, in cardiac arrest) I46.9, cardiac arrest, cause unspecified.

105. d. 93503, insertion and placement of flow directed catheter (eg. Swan-Ganz) for monitoring purposes.

106. d. 95811, polysomnography; sleep staging with 4 or more additional parameters of sleep, with initiation of continuous positive airway pressure (C-PAP) therapy or bi-level ventilation attended by a technologist, G47.33, obstructive sleep apnea (adult) (pediatric).

107. b. 90960, ESRD, for patients 20 years of age or older, N18.6, End stage renal failure, Chronic Kidney Disease.

108. c. 92928-RC, Modifier for right coronary artery, Transcatherter placement of an intracoronary stent(s). I25.10, Coronary atherosclerosis.

109. d. 95955, EEG during nonintracranial surgery (eg. Carotid surgery)

110. b. Dendrites are the afferent branches of the soma that receives signals.

111. b. Chronic. Atelectasis is the collapse of part or [much less commonly] all of a lung. A chronic form, designated middle lobe syndrome, results from compression of the middle lobe bronchus by surrounding lymph nodes.

112. d. Emphysema, a chronic pulmonary disease.

113. b. Osteosarcoma, a malignant sarcoma of the bone.

114. c. Chondrosarcoma a malignant tumor of the cartilage.

115. b. Pneumoconiosis; a condition of the respiratory tract due to inhalation of dust particles.

116. b. Empyema; a collection of pus in a body cavity (especially in the lung cavity).

117. a. Open, fracture of bone where broken end of bone had penetrated the skin.

118. a. Styloid.

119. c. Epiphyseal, means growth.

120. d. Interatrial, located between the atrial of the heart.

121. b. Nystagmus, movement may be in any direction. Etiology; may be congenital and in apparent to the patient; seen in bilateral amblyopia.

122. d. E. Coli; Escherichia coli.

123. b. Pituitary, also called the master gland.

124. b. H92.09: otogenic pain - of or originating within the ear, especially from inflammation of the ear. For H74.8x9 see Notes. Z18.81, retained glass fragments.

125. a. B20, HIV. I33.0 Acute and subacute infective endocarditis (use additional code to identify organism)

126. b. I48.91; unspecified atrial fibrillation, always code the reason for the encounter first. I42.8, other primary cardiomyopathies.

127. a. L02.432, B95.8; when coding L02 also identify the infective organism such as staphylococcus.

128. b. M48.02, M50.221, M50.222 mid-cervical region; keyword: displacement.

129. d. A41.2, R65.20, J96.00, K72.00; always code organism first then SIRS, followed by other manifestations.

130. d. Z23 is correct for influenza (flu), Z23 is the pneumococcal vaccine. R53.82 is chronic fatigue. J04.0 is acute laryngitis without mention of obstruction.

131. a. C91.11; key; in remission, B96.21: Shiga Toxin-producing Escherichia Coli [E coli] (STEC)

132. a. J15.0, Pneumonia due to Klebsiella pneumoniae ; J43.9, other emphysema; I49.8, other specified cardiac dysrhythmia; F06.8. Other specified mental disorders due to known physiological condition.

133. d. I20.0, Unstable angina; I10, Essential (primary) hypertension; I21.3, Acute myocardial infarction, episode of care unspecified; E11.69, Type 2 diabetes mellitus with other specified complication, code also the manifestation; I25.2, old myocardial infarction.

134. d. All of the Above. All codes are drug codes.

135. d. G0102, G0103; code digital rectal examination and prostate-specific antigen test. These are Medicare HCPC codes. Individual carriers may vary but coding exams are not reimbursement motivated.

136. c. G0130, code is a Medicare code. SEXA (Single energy x-ray absorptiometry bone density study).

137. d. G0108, code encounter for diabetes training.

138. c. G0008, G0009, code for each vaccination using Medicare payable codes.

139. b. Search for main terms and any applicable sub-terms.

140. a. Is considered to be an integral part of a larger service; these codes can stand alone and can only be coded with a larger procedure when done at another location deeming it completely separate and using a modifier 59 to get paid for it.

141. b. The code description has been revised.

142. a. They describe both physician and non-physician services. Category II and III CPT Codes are alphanumeric with a T or F at the end.

143. a. American Medical Association (AMA).

144. c. FI (and carriers); Fiscal Intermediary.

145. b. ALWAYS Check the tabular before assigning a code.

146. a. Code to the greatest detail.

147. c. Code both and sequence the acute (sub-acute) code first.

148. a. Must always be used as primary diagnosis.

149. c. COB; Coordination of Benefits.

150. a. Signs an agreement with the Fiscal Intermediary (FI).

151. d. All Patient Refined Diagnosis Related Groups (APR-DRGs)

152. d. Payment status indicator

153. b. A consultation

154. b. I23.8 Acute MI. An acute MI is considered to be anything under eight weeks duration from the time of initial onset. A chronic MI is considered anything over eight weeks with symptoms. An old MI is considered anything over eight weeks with NO symptoms.

155. c. Therapeutic procedure only

156. b. Excision of lesion; Full-thickness skin graft to scalp

157. d. Delirium tremens

158. c. Hypertensive cardiovascular disease with congestive heart failure. In order to use category I11 (Hypertensive heart disease) there must be a cause and effect relationship shown between the hypertension and the heart condition. "With" does not show this relationship nor does the fact that both conditions are listed on the same chart. The term "hypertensive" indicates a cause and effect relationship.

159. d. Centers for Medicare & Medicaid Services

160. b. Commission on Cancer of the American College of Surgeons

161. d. Promote national correct coding methodologies and reduce improper coding, with the overall goal of reducing improper payments of Medicare Part B and Medicaid claims.

162. d. All of the above might influence a facility's case mix

163. c. $40. Medicare pays 80% of $200, or $160, and the patient pays 20% of $200, or $40

164. c. David. The condition should be coded as a poisoning when there is an interaction of an over the counter drug and alcohol. Answers A, B & D are adverse effects of a correctly administered prescription drug.

165. b. The remittance advice

166. c. Prospective review.

167. c. Laser removal of condylomata

168. a. Tinnitus due to allergic reaction after administration of ear drops

169. b. A41.9, Sepsis, unspecified organism. R65.21, Severe sepsis with septic shock. N39.0, Urinary tract infection, site not specified. B96.21, Shiga toxin-producing Escherichia coli [E. coli] [STEC] O157 as the cause of diseases classified elsewhere. E86.0, Dehydration.

170. c. O03.1, Delayed or excessive hemorrhage following incomplete spontaneous abortion. 10D17ZZ, Extraction of Products of Conception, Retained, Via Natural or Artificial Opening.

171. a. Uniform Hospital Discharge Data Set (UHDDS). The definitions in the UHDDS should be followed to sequence codes for reporting inpatient information to third party payers.

172. d. Firewalls

173. d. 99203-32. Office or other outpatient visit for the evaluation and management of a new patient, which requires a medically appropriate history and/or examination and low level of medical decision making. When using time for code selection, 30-44 minutes of total time is spent on the date of the encounter.

174. c. K40.20, Bilateral inguinal hernia, without obstruction or gangrene, not specified as recurrent. 0YUA0JZ, Supplement Bilateral Inguinal Region with Synthetic Substitute, Open Approach.

175. d. 29881-LT, Arthroscopy, knee, surgical; with meniscectomy (medial OR lateral, including any meniscal shaving) including debridement/shaving of articular cartilage (chondroplasty), same or separate compartment(s), when performed. 29874-LT, Arthroscopy, knee, surgical; for removal of loose body or foreign body (eg, osteochondritis dissecans fragmentation, chondral fragmentation).

176. a. Database.

177. a. Doctors' progress note section. The physician releasing the patient should write a final note of summary of the patient's course of treatment, stating the patient's condition at discharge, and instructions for the patient's activity, diet and medications as well as any follow up appoints or instructions. If a patient expires, the final notes describe the circumstances regarding the death, the findings, the cause of death, and whether or not an autopsy was performed.

178. c. Used and sequenced as a secondary diagnosis.

179. a. 63005, Laminectomy with exploration and/or decompression of spinal cord and/or cauda equina, without facetectomy, foraminotomy or discectomy (eg, spinal stenosis), 1 or 2 vertebral segments; lumbar, except for spondylolisthesis.

180. b. H66.93, 69433, 69433. Since the procedure is bilateral, either code twice or use the modifier -50.

181. c. Z38.00, Q37.9. procedure codes are not assigned unless there is documentation that a procedure was performed.

182. d. Osteoporosis

183. c. A surgical operation is one or more surgical procedures performed at one time for one patient using a common approach or for a common purpose.

184. b. G56.00, Carpal tunnel syndrome, unspecified upper limb. 64721, Neuroplasty and/or transposition; median nerve at carpal tunnel.

185. d. 49501, Repair initial inguinal hernia, age 6 months to younger than 5 years, with or without hydrocelectomy; incarcerated or strangulated.

186. c. J96.00, Acute respiratory failure, unspecified whether with hypoxia or hypercapnia. I50.20, Unspecified systolic (congestive) heart failure. 5A1945Z, Respiratory Ventilation, 24-96 Consecutive Hours. 0BH17EZ, Insertion of Endotracheal Airway into Trachea, Via Natural or Artificial Opening.

187. b. N39.3, 51990. N39.3 covers stress incontinence in both female and male in ICD-10.

188. c. Is a system for documenting the extent or spread of cancer. Staging is a term used to refer to the progression of cancer. In accessing most types of cancer a method (staging) is used to determine how far the cancer has progressed. The cancer is described in terms of how large the main tumor is, the degree to which it has invaded surrounding tissue, and the extent to which it has spread to lymph glands or other areas of the body. Staging not only helps to assess outlook but also the most appropriate treatment.

189. d. Low forceps. To use code O80 the delivery has to require minimal or no assistance, with or without episiotomy, without fetal manipulation [e.g., rotation version] or instrumentation [forceps] of a spontaneous, cephalic, vaginal, full-term, single, live-born infant.

190. c. H26.9, 66984-LT. Subconjunctival injections are included in 66984

191. a. 33430. Valvuloplasty is a plastic repair of a valve

192. a. Primipara

193. d. Acronyms. An acronym is a word formed from the initial letters of the major parts of a compound term.

194. a. Z51.11, C50.919. The cancer is coded as a current condition as long as patient is receiving adjunct therapy.

195. c. N21.1, 0T7D0DZ. N21.1 is Calculus in urethra and 0T7D0DZ is Dilation of Urethra with Intraluminal Device, Open Approach.

196. b. I21.3, J44.9 , I50.20, I10, I48.91. Z90.89 acquired absence of organ is intended to be used for patient care where the absence of an organ affects treatment.

197. c. Is also known as genital warts

198. a. 60520.Thymectomy, partial or total; transcervical approach (separate procedure).

199. c. Taylor

200. d. 90471, 90723. If the immunization is the only service that the patient receives, two codes are used to report the service: the immunization administration code is first and then the code for the vaccine/toxoid.

Mock Exam #3 - 100 Questions

201. A man suffered a severe crushing injury to his left upper leg. Two days after surgery, the doctor completed a dressing change under general anesthesia. How would you report this service?

a. 16020-LT
b. 15852, 01232, J2060
c. 01232-P6
d. 15852-LT

202. Dr. Jess removed a 4.5 cm (excised diameter) cystic lesion from Amy's forehead. The ulcerated lesion was anesthetized with 20 mg of 1% Lidocaine and then elliptically excised. The wound was closed with a layered suture technique and a sterile dressing applied. The wound closure, according to Dr. Jess's documentation, was 5.3 cm. How would you report this procedure?

a. 11446, 12053-51
b. 11646, 12013-51
c. 11446, J2001 x 2, 12013-59
d. 11313, 12053-59

203. Martha has a non-healing wound on the tip of her nose. After an evaluation by Dr. Martino, a dermatologist, Martha is scheduled for a procedure the following week. Dr. Martino documented an autologous split thickness skin graft to the tip of Martha's nose. A simple debridement of granulated tissues is completed prior to the placement. Using a dermatome, a split thickness skin graft was harvested from the left thigh. The graft is placed onto the nose defect and secured with sutures. The donor site is examined, which confirms good hemostasis. How would you report this procedure?

a. 99213-25, 15050
b. 15050, 15004, 15005-59
c. 15277, 11042-59
d. 15120

204. Code for a breast biopsy, two lesions, with placement of breast clip, with imaging of the specimen; includes ultrasound guidance.

a. 19081, 19084
b. 19083 X 2
c. 19083, 19084
d. 19084, 19085

205. Dr. Alexis completed Mohs surgery on Ralph's left arm. She reported routine stains on all slides, mapping, and color coding of specimens. The procedure was accomplished in three stages with a total of seven blocks in the second stage. How would you report Dr. Alexis' services?

a. 17313, 17314-58, 17315-59, 88314-59
b. 17311, 17312 x 7
c. 17313, 17314 x 2, 17315 x 2
d. 17311, 88302, 17314 x 3, 17312 x 7

206. How should you code an excision of a lesion when completed with an adjacent tissue transfer or rearrangement?

a. The excision is always reported in addition to the adjacent tissue transfer or rearrangement.

b. The excision is not separately reported with adjacent tissue transfer or rearrangement codes.

c. Code only malignant lesions in addition to the adjacent tissue transfer or rearrangement codes.

d. Code the lesion with a modifier -51 and code in addition to the adjacent tissue transfer or rearrangement codes.

207. Tina fell from a step ladder while clearing drain gutters at her home. She suffered contusions and multiple lacerations. At the emergency room she received sutures for lacerations to her arm, hand, and foot. The doctor completed the following repairs: superficial repair to the arm of 12.8 cm, a single-layered closure of 7.9 cm that required extensive cleaning and removal of glass from the hand, and a simple repair to the foot of 9.6 cm How would you report the wound repairs?

a. 12034, 12036, 12046, 12007
b. 12006, 12034-59
c. 12044, 12006-51
d. 12005, 12004 x 2

208. The 18-year old patient presented for an annual well visit and NorPlant implantable contraceptive capsule. The chief complaint was "annual exam." On the form the provider checked detailed Hx, detailed exam and Low Medical Decision Making.

a. 99213
b. 99214, 11981
c. 99395, 11981
d. 11981

209. James had a malignant lesion removed from his right arm (excised diameter 4.6 cm). During the same visit the dermatologist noticed a new growth on James' left arm. Dr. Terry took a biopsy of the new lesion and sent it in for pathology. The biopsy site required a simple closure. How would Dr. Terry report the biopsy procedure (assuming two procedures were reported)?

a. The biopsy is included in the primary procedure and not reported
b. 11106-59
c. 11406, 11106-59
d. 11106, 12001, 11406-51

210. Sally suffered a burst fracture to her lumbar spine during a skiing accident. Dr. Phyllis performed a partial corpectomy to L2 by a transperitoneal approach followed by anterior arthrodesis of L1-L3. She also positioned anterior instrumentation and placed a structural allograft to L1-L3. How would Dr. Phyllis report this procedure?

a. 63090, 22558-51, 22585, 22845, 20931
b. 63085, 22533, 22585-51, 22808-59
c. 22612 x 2, 22808, 22840-51, 20931
d. 22585, 22585-51, 22845-51, 20931-59

211. A patient suffered a fracture of the femur head. He had an open treatment of the femoral head with a replacement using a Medicon alloy femoral head and methylmethacrylate cement. How would you report this procedure?

a. 27236
b. 27235
c. 27238
d. 27275, 27236-59

212. What modifier should you report when the same physician provided a re-reduction of a fracture?

a. 76
b. 59
c. 77
d. 54

213. A patient suffered a penetrating knife wound to his back. A surgeon performed wound exploration with enlargement of the site, debridement, and removal of gravel from the site. The surgeon decided a laparotomy procedure was not necessary at this time. How would you report this procedure?

a. This procedure is bundled with the laparotomy
b. 49000, 97602-51, 20100-59
c. 49000, 20102-59
d. 20102

214. While playing at home, Riley dislocated his patella, when he fell from a tree. The surgeon documented an open dislocation. Riley underwent a closed treatment under anesthesia. How would you report the treatment and diagnoses?

a. 27420, S83.006A
b. 27562, S83.006A, W14.XXXA , Y92.099
c. 27840, 27562-51, S83.006A, W14.XXXA
d. 27562, S83.006A

215. Sarah presented to her primary care physician with pain and swelling in the right elbow. After careful examination he referred her to an orthopedic surgeon for a second opinion. Dr. Femur diagnosed Sarah with acute osteomyelitis of the olecranon process and recommended surgery. Sarah agreed to the surgery and underwent a sequestrectomy, through a posterior incision, with a loose repair over drains ending the procedure. Dr. Femur sent a written report back to Sarah's primary care physician along with the operative report. How would you report the procedure?

a. 99244-57, 24138-RT
b. 99214, 99244-57
c. 24138-RT
d. 99214, 23172-59

216. Code for a revision of total shoulder arthroplasty, including allograft when performed; humeral AND glenoid component.

a. 23472
b. 23473
c. 23474
d. 29827

217. Mike had a bicycle accident and suffered deep hematomas in both knees. He underwent a bilateral incision and drainage. How would you report the procedure?

a. 27301-50
b. 10040
c. 27303
d. 27301-59

218. A patient had a unilateral percutaneous intradiscal annuloplasty (IDET) using radio frequency energy on L3-L5 with magnetic resonance guidance for needle placement. How would you report this professional service procedure?

a. 22526, 22527, 77002-26
b. 22526, 22527, 77021-26
c. 22899, 77021-26
d. 22526, 77021-26

219. What modifier is exempt from the following codes: 20974, 61107, 93602, 94610?

a. RT and LT
b. 63
c. 59
d. 51

220. Code for the removal of a subcutaneous 3 cm tumor from the soft tissue of the right hip.

a. 27043
b. 27043-RT
c. 27047
d. 27047-RT

221. What code would you report for a cervical approach of a mediastinotomy with exploration, drainage, removal of foreign body, or biopsy?

a. 39010
b. 39000
c. 39200
d. 39401

222. Roger had a rhinoplasty to correct damage caused by a broken nose. One year later he had a secondary rhinoplasty with major revisions. At the end of the second surgery the incisions were closed with a single layer technique. How would you report the second procedure?

a. 30450
b. 30450-78
c. 30420, 12014
d. 30430, 12014-59

223. A surgeon started with a diagnostic thoracoscopy. During the same surgical session she completed a surgical thoracoscopy to control a hemorrhage. How would you report this procedure?

a. 32601
b. 32601, 32654-59
c. 32505
d. 32654

224. Dr. Sacra performed a CABG surgery on Fred five months ago. Today, Dr. Sacra completed another coronary artery bypass using three venous grafts with harvesting of a femoropopliteal vein segment. How would Dr. Sacra report her work for the current surgery?

a. 33512, 33530-51, 35572-51
b. 33535, 35500-51, 33519
c. 33512, 33530, 35572
d. 33535, 33519, 33530-51, 35500

225. What do the primary codes 33880 and 33881 include?

a. Placement of all distal extensions, if required.
b. Placement of all proximal extensions in the thoracic aorta
c. Repair of extensions in the thoracic aorta
d. Repositioning of all leads and extensions in the thoracic aorta

226. Mrs. Reyes had a temporary ventricular pacemaker placed at the start of a procedure. This temporary system was used as support during the procedure only. How would you report the temporary system?

a. 33210
b. 33211
c. 33207
d. 33210, 33207-51, 33235-51

227. Mr. Azeri, a 68-year-old patient, has a dual-chamber pacemaker. The leads in this system were recalled. The leads were extracted via transvenous technique, the generator was left in place, and new leads were inserted via transvenous technique. How would you report this procedure?

a. 33214, 33215-51, 33208-51, 33218-51
b. 33215, 33210-51, 33216-51
c. 33208, 33235-51, 33217-51
d. 33235, 33217-51

228. A 35-year-old female patient with a venous catheter requires a blood sample for hematology testing. The sample is collected via her PICC catheter. How would you report this procedure?

a. 36415
b. 36592
c. 36591
d. 37799

229. A patient underwent a secondary percutaneous transluminal thrombectomy for retrieval of a short segment of embolus evident during another percutaneous intervention procedure. How would you report this secondary procedure?

a. 37184, 37186
b. 37186 in addition to the primary procedure
c. 37185, 76000
d. 37187

230. Lynn has a family history of colon cancer and is scheduled for a screening colonoscopy. During the procedure, three polyps were discovered and removed via hot biopsy forceps technique. The polyps were reported as benign. What diagnoses and procedure(s) codes capture these services?

a. Z12.11, Z80.0, 45315, 45331
b. Z12.11, D12.6, Z80.0, 45384
c. 45378
d. 45378, 45384

231. Dr. Blue performs a secondary closure of the abdominal wall for evisceration (outside the postoperative period). He opens the former incision and removes the remaining sutures; necrotic fascia is debrided down to viable tissue. The abdominal wall is then closed with sutures. How would you report the closure?

a. 11043
b. This is a bundled procedure and not reported
c. 39541
d. 49900

232. Heather lost her teeth following a motorcycle accident. She underwent a posterior, bilateral vestibuloplasty, which allows her to wear complete dentures. How would you report this procedure?

a. 40845, 15002
b. 40843-50
c. 40844
d. 40843

233. Dr. Erin is treating a 58-year-old male patient with a history of chewing tobacco. Dr. Erin finds a 3.4 cm tumor at the base of his tongue. She places needles under fluoroscopic guidance for sub-sequential interstitial radioelement application. How would you report the professional services?

a. 41019, 77002-26
b. 41019, 77012-26, 77021-26
c. 61770, 41019-59
d. 77002

234. An 88-year-old male patient suffering from dementia accidentally pulled out his gastrostomy tube during the night. Dr. Keys, an interventional radiologist, takes him into an angiography suite, administers moderate sedation (an independent observer was present during the procedure), probes the site with a catheter and injects contrast medium for assessment and tube placement. Dr. Keys finds that the entry site remains open and replaced the tube into the proper position. The intra-service time for the procedure took 45 minutes. How would Dr. Keys report his services?

a. 49440, 99155, 99156
b. 49440, 49450-59
c. 49450, 99152, 99153
d. 49450

235. Katherine had a hernioplasty to repair a recurrent ventral incarcerated hernia with implantation of mesh for closure. The surgeon completed debridement for necrotizing soft tissue due to infection. Total length of defect 6 cm. How would you report this procedure?

a. 49616, 11005-51, 49594
b. 49615, 11005-51, 49594
c. 49615
d. 49525, 11006, 49594-51

236. A 28-year-old patient underwent a proctosigmoidoscopy with ablation of five tumors under moderate sedation. The same provider performed the procedure and the sedation. The intra- service time for the procedure was 30 minutes. How would you report this procedure?

a. 45320-P1
b. 45320 x 5
c. 45320
d. 45320, 99152

237. Harry had a sphincterotomy and an ERCP with a stent placed into the bile duct. How would you report this procedure?

a. 43274
b. 43262
c. 43260, 43274
d. 43264

238. The ER doctor performed peritoneal lavage, an abdominal X-ray (single view) and an EPF History and Exam and Moderate MDM encounter.

a. 99283, 43753, 74018
b. 99284, 44701, 74018
c. 99283, 49084, 74018
d. 99284, 49329, 74018

239. Sharon had a laparoscopic cholecystectomy with cholangiography. How would you report this procedure?

a. 47605, 47570-59
b. 47605
c. 47563
d. 47579

240. A patient had a renal auto-transplantation extracorporeal surgery, reimplantation of a kidney, and a partial nephrectomy. How would you report this procedure?

a. 50340, 50380, 50240-51
b. 50543, 50370-52
c. 50380, 50240-51
d. 50380, 50240-59

241. Bill, a 52-year-old male patient, was admitted to the hospital and treated for prostatic malignancy. His doctor dictated a detailed history, detailed exam, and straightforward medical decision-making for admission. He was treated with interstitial transperineal prostate brachytherapy, including implantation of 51 iodine-125 seeds. His doctor visited him the day after the procedure. How would you report the professional service by the therapeutic radiologist who did both the implantation and brachytherapy?

a. 99222, 55876, 77763 x 51
b. 55875, 77778
c. 99221, 58720, 77770
d. 58346, 77799 x 125

242. Harry had a couple of stones in both kidneys. He was taken into the lithotripsy unit and placed on the lithotripsy table in a supine position with the induction of anesthesia. The stones were well visualized and the patient received a total of 3,500 shocks with a maximum power setting of 3.0. The treatment was successful. How would you report this procedure?

a. 50590
b. 50561
c. 50060
d. 50080

243. Tom was placed under general anesthesia (by an anesthesiologist) for an excision of a local lesion of the epididymis. How would you report the surgeon's services?

a. 54861-50
b. 54860-47
c. 54830, 00920-51
d. 54830

244. Alex suffered several injuries to his upper leg muscles and penis when he fell onto the bar of his touring bicycle. The day of the accident, Dr. Green completed muscle repair surgery to Alex's upper legs. Today, three days after the leg surgeries, Dr. Green took Alex back to the operating suite to complete an unrelated repair to the penis. Dr. Green completed a plastic repair to correct the penal injury. What code(s) would capture today's procedure?

a. 54440-79
b. 27385, 54440-59
c. 54620-79
d. 54440-26

245. Heather had a bilateral laparoscopic occlusion of her fallopian tubes using a Falope ring. How would you report this procedure?

a. 58615
b. 58671
c. 58671-50
d. 58679-50

246. A 65-year-old male patient has an indwelling nephroureteral double-J stent tube replaced to treat a ureteral obstruction caused by a stricture from postoperative scarring. His stent tube is exchanged every two months to prevent occlusion in the stent, UTI, and loss of kidney function. Dr. Mott did this procedure via a transurethral approach under conscious sedation and provided the radiological supervision and interpretation. How would you report this procedure?

a. 50605, 50382
b. 50385, 52283, 99151
c. 50385
d. 50386

247. Dr. Blue provided interpretation and results for a needle electromyography for anal sphincter function. How would you report this service?

a. 51784
b. 51784, 51785-51
c. 55875
d. 51785-26

248. A 48-year-old patient with BPH has his prostate removed via a laser enucleation. During this procedure he also has a vasectomy. What code(s) would report this procedure?

a. 52648
b. 52649
c. 52649, 55250-51
d. 52647

249. What code series would you refer to for patients who have had a previous cesarean delivery and now present with the expectation of a vaginal delivery?

a. 59400 - 59140
b. 59618 - 59622
c. 59610 - 59614
d. 59610 - 59622

250. The procedure was a vaginal colpopexy to reposition the patient's vagina. Approach was intra-peritoneal. During the procedure, the vagina was sutured to the sacrospinous ligament to secure it in place.

a. 57283, 57556
b. 57283, 58263, 58292
c. 57283, 58263
d. None of the answers are correct

251. An infant born at 33 weeks underwent five photocoagulation treatments to both eyes due to retinopathy of prematurity at six months of age. The physician used an operating microscope during these procedures. These treatments occurred once per day for a defined treatment period of five days. How would you report all of these services?

a. 67229 -50
b. 67229 x 5
c. 67229, 69990
d. 67229

252. Todd had a tumor removed from his left temporal bone. How would you report this service?

a. 61563
b. 61500
c. 69979, 69990-51
d. 69970

253. Jennifer was admitted to the hospital for an aspiration of two thyroid cysts. Her physician completed this procedure with CT guidance of the needle including interpretation and report. How would you report the professional services?

a. 60300-26, 76942-26
b. 60300 x 2, 77012-26
c. 10021, 60300-51, 77012-26
d. 60300

254. Baby Smith was diagnosed with meningitis. His physician placed a needle through the fontanel at the suture line to obtain a spinal fluid sample on Monday. The needle was withdrawn and the area bandaged. The baby required another subdural tap bilaterally on Wednesday. How would you report Wednesday's service?

a. 61001
b. 61000, 61001
c. 61070
d. 61001-50

255. Max had a bilateral revision fenestration operation. How would you report this procedure?

a. 69949
b. 69949-50
c. 69930
d. 69915

256. Dr. Martin performed an excision at the middle cranial fossa for a vascular lesion. This procedure was completed in an intradural fashion with dural repair and graft. His partner, Dr. Sutter, performed an infratemporal approach with decompression of the auditory canal. How should Dr. Martin report her services?

a. 61590, 61606-51
b. 61606-62
c. 61606
d. 61601

257. After a snow skiing accident, Barry had a cervical laminoplasty to four vertebral segments. How should you report this procedure?

a. 63050 x 4
b. 22600, 63051-51
c. 22842, 63045, 63050
d. 63050

258. How is a neuroplasty procedure described in the CPT Professional Edition?

a. The decompression or freeing of intact nerve from scar tissue, including external neurolysis and/or transposition
b. The surgical repair of nerves using only microscopic techniques
c. The position of nerves tested one or more anatomic digits
d. The decompression or freeing of an intact vein from scar tissue, including external neurolysis and/or transposition

259. Phyllis fell down on the ice and fractured her leg. The fall also caused severe injury to the muscles and tore several nerves. Her physician completed suturing of two major peripheral nerves in her leg without transposition and shortened the bone. After the surgery she was seen by a physical therapist for ongoing treatment and gait training. How would you report the surgical procedure?

a. 64857, 64859-51, 64876-51
b. 64856, 64857
c. 64857, 64859, 64876
d. 64858, 64857, 64859, 64876

260. John was hospitalized for a repair of a laceration to his left conjunctiva by mobilization and rearrangement. How should you report this procedure?

a. 65273-LT
b. 67930
c. 65272
d. 67930-LT

261. How does the CPT Professional Edition define a new patient?

a. A new patient is one who has not received any professional services from the physician or another physician of the same specialty who belongs to the same group practice, within the past two years.

b. A new patient is one who has not received any professional services from the physician or another physician of the same specialty who belongs to the same group practice, within the past three years.

c. A new patient is one who has received professional services from the physician or another physician of the same specialty within the last two years for the same problem.

d. A new patient is one who has received hospital services but has never been seen in the clinic by the reporting physician.

262. James, a 35-year-old new patient, received 45 minutes of counseling and risk factor reduction intervention services from Dr. Kelly. Dr. Kelly talked to James about how to avoid sports injuries. Currently, James does not have any symptoms or injuries and wants to maintain this status. This was the only service rendered. How would you report this service?

a. 99213
b. 99203
c. 99385
d. 99403

263. Andrea, a 52-year-old patient, had a hysterectomy on Monday morning. That afternoon, after returning to her hospital room, she suffered a cardiac arrest. A cardiologist responded to the call and delivered one hour and 35 minutes of critical care. During this time the cardiologist ordered a single view chest x-ray and provided ventilation management. How should you report the cardiologist's services?

a. 99291, 99292
b. 99291, 99292, 71045, 94002
c. 71045, 94002, 99231
d. 99291, 99292, 99292-52

264. Brandon was seen in Dr. Shaw's office after falling off his bunk bed. Brandon's mother reported that Brandon and his sister were jumping on the beds when she heard a "thud." Brandon complained of knee pain and had trouble walking. Dr. Shaw ordered a knee x-ray that was done at the imaging center across the street. The x-ray showed no fracture or dislocations. Dr. Shaw had seen Brandon for his school physical six months ago. Today, Dr. Shaw documented a detailed examination and decision-making of moderate complexity. He also instructed Brandon's mother that if Brandon had any additional pain or trouble walking he should see an orthopedic specialist. How should Dr. Shaw report her services from today's visit?

a. 99204
b. 99394, 99214
c. 99214
d. 99203

265. Adam, a 48-year-old patient, presented to Dr. Crampon's office with complaints of fever, malaise, chills, chest pain, and a severe cough. Dr. Crampon took a history, did an exam, and ordered a chest x-ray. After reviewing the x-ray, Dr. Crampon admitted Adam to the hospital for treatment of pneumonia. After his regular office hours, Dr. Crampon visited Adam in the hospital where he dictated a comprehensive history, comprehensive examination, and decision-making of moderate complexity. How would you report Dr. Crampon's services?

a. 99214
b. 99222
c. 99204, 99222-51
d. 99223, 99214-21

266. Which below are not included with subsequent intensive care codes 99478-99480?

a. Cardiac and respiratory monitoring
b. Vital sign monitoring
c. Enteral nutritional adjustments
d. None of the answers are correct

267. Larry is being managed for his warfarin therapy on an outpatient basis. Dr. Nancy continues to review Larry's INR tests, gives patient instructions, dosage adjustment as needed, and ordered additional tests. How would you report the initial 90 days of therapy including 8 INR measurements?

a. 93793
b. 93793, 99471
c. 99214
d. This services is bundled with evaluation and management services

268. Dr. Jane admitted a 67-year-old woman to the coronary care unit for an acute myocardial infarction. The admission included a comprehensive history, comprehensive examination, and high complexity decision-making. Dr. Jane visited the patient on days two and three and documented (each day) an expanded problem focused examination and decision-making of moderate complexity. On day four, Dr. Jane moved the patient to the medical floor and documented a problem focused examination and straight forward decision-making. Day five, Dr. Jane discharged the patient to home. The discharge took over an hour. How would you report the services from day one to day five?

a. 99213, 99232, 99231, 99239 x 2
b. 99221, 99222, 99223, 99238
c. 99231, 99232, 99417, 99238
d. 99223, 99232, 99232, 99231, 99239

269. The provider performed a 120 minute E & M service of a critically ill neonate plus selective head hypothermia reported as two days.

a. 99291, 99184
b. 99292 x 4, 99184
c. 99291 x 2, 99184 x 1
d. 99291, 99292 x 2, 99184

270. Mr. Johnson, a 38-year-old established patient is being seen for management of his hypertension, diabetes, and weight control. On his last visit, he was told he had a diabetic foot ulcer and needed to be hospitalized for this condition. He decided to get a second opinion and went to see Dr. Myers. This was the first time Dr. Myers had seen Mr. Johnson. Dr. Myers documented a comprehensive history, comprehensive examination, and decision-making of high complexity. He concurred with hospitalization for the foot ulcer and sent a report back to Mr. Johnson's primary care doctor. How would you report Dr. Myers visit?

a. 99245
b. 99205
c. 99215
d. 99255

271. Code for the supervision by a control physician of inter-facility transport care of the critically ill or critically injured pediatric patient, 24 months of age or younger, includes two-way communication with transport team before transport, at the referring facility and during the transport, including data interpretation and report; first 30 minutes:

a. 99485
b. 99486
c. 99487
d. 99489

272. Lucas, a three-year-old new patient is seen for a well-child examination. The doctor documents an age appropriate history, examination, anticipatory guidelines, risk factor reduction intervention, and indicates Lucas' immunizations are up to date. How would you report this service?

a. 99392
b. 99213-25, 99385
c. 99203
d. 99382

273. An anesthesiologist provides general anesthesia for a 72-year-old patient with mild systemic disease who is undergoing a ventral hernia repair. How would you report the anesthesia service?

a. 00834-P2, 99100
b. 00832-P2, 99100
c. 49591, 00834, 99100-P2
d. 00832

274. Dr. Warren performed a transesophageal echocardiography for a congenital cardiac condition on a 16-year-old patient. Prior to the probe placement, moderate conscious sedation was administered. The probe was placed, images acquired, interpretation and reports were completed in the provider's office. This procedure lasted 45 minutes. What code(s) capture the services performed by Dr. Warren?

a. 93315, 99152, 99153
b. 00320, 99152, 99153
c. 93315
d. 93315-P1

275. Katherine is a 77-year-old patient with a severe hypertensive disease. She underwent a cataract surgery to both eyes under general anesthesia. Dr. Sharon, the anesthesiologist, performed the anesthesia. Prior to induction of anesthesia Dr. Sharon completed a preoperative visit and documented a detailed history, detailed examination, and low complexity decision- making on this new patient. How would you report Dr. Sharon's services?

a. 99203, 00142-P2, 99100
b. 66820, 00144
c. 00140-P1, 99116-59
d. 00142-P3, 99100

276. A surgeon performed a cervical approach esophagoplasty with repair of a tracheosophageal fistula under general anesthesia. The surgeon performed both the procedure and the anesthesia. How would you report these services?

a. 00500, 43305
b. 43305-47
c. 00500-47
d. Both A and C

277. Which service is not included with anesthesia services?

a. Swan-Ganz monitoring
b. Administration of blood
c. Blood pressure
d. Mass spectrometry

278. A patient was placed under general anesthesia for a simple incision and removal of a foreign body from the subcutaneous tissue. This procedure usually requires local anesthesia. Due to unusual circumstances, which required general anesthesia, what modifier would best describe this situation?

a. 47
b. 22
c. 23
d. P6

279. Erin, a 45-year-old, asymptomatic female comes in for her annual bilateral screening mammography. Her physician ordered a computer aided detection along with the mammography. The procedure was performed in a hospital. How would you report the professional services for this study?

a. 77067-26,
b. 77066-26, 77065-26-59
c. 77047-26, 77067-51
d. 77067, 77053-51

280. A patient presents to a freestanding radiology center and had ultrasonic guidance needle placement with imaging supervision and interpretation of two separate lesions in the left breast. The procedure required several passes to complete. How would you report the imaging procedure?

a. 33016 x 2
b. 76941
c. 76942 x 2-LT
d. 76942-LT

281. Sally had a DXA bone density study for her hips, pelvis, and spine. The procedure was performed in a hospital. How would you report for the professional services of this study?

a. 77078-26, 77080-26
b. 77080-26
c. 77086-26
d. 77081-26, 77080-26

282. Which of the following tests is not part of a liver panel?

a. Bilirubin
b. Albumin
c. Alkaline phosphatase
d. Creatinine

283. Rheumatoid arthritis typically affects the

a. Intervertebral disks
b. Hips and shoulders
c. Knees and small joints of the hands and feet
d. Large, weight-bearing joints

284. "Pill-rolling" tremor is a characteristic symptom of

a. Epilepsy
b. Myasthenia gravis
c. Guillain Barre syndrome
d. Parkinson disease

285. A seventy-five year old female was admitted for repair of a hiatal hernia which was performed on the first day of admission. While recovering, the patient fell out of her bed and sustained a fractured femur which was surgically reduced. Further complications included severe angina for which a cardiac catheterization and PTCA were performed. The principal procedure is:

a. Femur reduction
b. Herniorrhaphy
c. Catheterization
d. PTCA

286. A patient is on Coumadin therapy. Which of the following tests is commonly ordered to monitor the patient's Coumadin levels?

a. Bleeding time
b. Blood smear
c. Partial thromboplastin time
d. Prothrombin time

287. Which of the following is a congenital condition that is the most severe neural tube defect?

a. Meningeocele
b. Myelominingocele
c. Spina bifida occulta
d. Severe combined immunodeficiency

288. The hypothalamus, thalamus and pituitary gland are all parts of the _________.

a. Brain stem
a. Cerebellum
c. Cerebrum
d. Limbic system

289. Myringoplasty

a. 69620
b. 69635
c. 69610
d. 69420

290. Patient with a traumatic rupture of the ear drum repaired the tympanoplasty with incision of the mastoid. Repair of ossicular chain not required.

a. 69641
b. 69646
c. 69642
d. 69635

291. Which modifier would you use to report with code 88239 if the test was looking for hereditary breast cancer?

a. OB
b. 59
c. 91
d. OA

292. Marvin had a breath alcohol test completed at the hospital after the police arrested him for racing his four-wheeler past a McDonald's drive through window. Marvin's breath alcohol test was mathematically calculated. How would you report the calculation on this test?

a. 82075
b. 82075 x 2
c. 82075, 82355
d. 82355

293. Dr. Monday provided a comprehensive clinical pathology consultation at the request of Dr. Adams. This request was regarding a patient with various infections, drug allergies, skin rash, and Down's syndrome. The patient is in the hospital intensive care unit being treated with intravenous antibiotics. Dr. Monday did not see the patient but he reviewed the patient's history, highly complex medical records, and provided a written report back to Dr. Adams regarding his findings and recommendations for further treatment. How would Dr. Monday report his services?

a. 80505
b. 99244
c. 99244-25, 80503
d. 99255-25, 80506

294. A patient had a semi-quantitative urinalysis for infectious agent detection. How should you report this test?

a. 81050
b. 81005
c. 81007
d. 81005, 83518

295. Code 3011F describes which diagnostic or screening process?

a. Lipid panel results including total cholesterol, HDL-C, triglycerides, calculated LDL-C
b. Lipid panel results including total cholesterol
c. Lipid panel results including cholesterol, triglycerides, lipoprotein
d. Lipid panel results including cholesterol, triglycerides, carbon dioxide, glucose, potassium

296. A 58-year-old male patient with abdominal pain and episodes of bright red blood in his stool reports to his physician's office for a check-up. His physician performs a digital rectal exam and tests for occult blood. Dr. Smith documents this blood occult test was done for purposes other than colorectal cancer screening. How would you report the occult blood test?

a. 82270
b. 82274
c. 82271
d. 82272

297. Kathy has had intermittent abdominal pain, occasional diarrhea, stool frequency, and bloating. Her symptoms have worsened over the past two months. Her physician orders a fecal Calprotectin test to check for Crohn's disease. How should you report the lab test?

a. 82270
b. 82272, 83993
c. 83993
d. 82271, 82272

298. Colin had a comprehensive audiometry threshold evaluation and speech recognition testing to the left ear. What code(s) capture this procedure?

a. 92557-52
b. 92553, 92556
c. 92557
d. 92700-59

299. An adult patient had the following immunizations with administration: yellow fever vaccine, subcutaneous injection, Hepatitis B vaccine IM injection, Plague vaccine, Intramuscular injection. How would you report these services?

a. 90460, 90461 x 2, 90717-51, 90746-51, 90691-51
b. 90471, 90472 x 2, 90717, 90746, 90691
c. 90473, 90474 x 2, 90746, 90691, 90717
d. 90471, 90472 x 2, 90691-51, 90746-51, 90717-51

300. Sally suffered from dehydration after running a marathon. She was taken into her primary care doctor's office. Dr. Small checked Sally and ordered hydration therapy with normal saline. The hydration lasted 45 minutes. How would you report this service?

a. 96365
b. 96360, 96361
c. 96360
d. 96369, 96370

Mock Exam #3 - Answers and Rationale

201. d. 15852-LT. The code 15852 includes “under anesthesia (other than local).” You can find this code in the index of the CPT Professional Edition under Dressing, Change, and Anesthesia. Modifier -LT provides additional information regarding which side of the body was involved in the procedure.

202. a. 11446, 12053-51. You would report this excision to a benign lesion. In the CPT Professional Edition under the heading Excision – Benign Lesions, cystic lesion is given as an example, (layered) intermediate closure should be reported in addition to the excision. The local anesthesia is included per the CPT Surgery section guidelines.

203. d. 15120. This is an autograft (coming from one part of a patient’s body to another). In the CPT Professional Edition under the Skin Replacement Surgery and Skin Substitutes subsection in the Surgery/Integumentary System (15002–15278), the guidelines state, “Procedures are coded by recipient site,” [which is the nose in this question], further, the guidelines read, “…includes simple debridement of granulation tissue.” There is no documentation of an additional office visit on the day of the procedure.

204. c. 19083, 19084. 19083: Biopsy, breast, with placement of breast localization device(s) (eg, clip, metallic pellet), when performed, and imaging of the biopsy specimen, when performed, percutaneous; first lesion, including; ultrasound guidance; 19084, second code is add-on for second lesion. AMA guidelines “Use 19084 in conjunction with 19083”.

205. c. 17313, 17314 x 2, 17315 x 2. Mohs surgery is reported by anatomic site. The code description includes mapping, color coding of specimens, and routine stains. The first stage is reported with code 17313, the two additional stages are reported with 17314 x 2, and the additional blocks in stage two are reported with code 17315 x 2.

206. b. The excision is not separately reported with adjacent tissue transfer or rearrangement codes. The CPT Professional Edition subcategory guidelines for Adjacent Tissue Transfer or Rearrangement procedures under the Surgery/ Integumentary System, state, “excision (including lesion).”

207. c. 12044, 12006-51. In the CPT Professional Edition under the heading for Repair (Closure), the guidelines define simple, intermediate, and complex. The repair to the arm and foot are classified to simple repairs and reported by the sum of lengths of repairs for each group of anatomic site, 12006. The repair to the hand is classified as intermediate (refer to the definitions) 12044. These guidelines also state, under number two, multiple wounds, "When more than one classification of wounds is repaired, list the more complicated as the primary procedure and the less complicated as the secondary procedure, using modifier -51."

208. c. 99395, 11981. If the chief complaint is "annual visit" this should be reported as a preventive medicine visit. The notes in CPT under 11971 and 11976 direct the coder to report 11981 for the insertion of non-biodegradable drug delivery implants. Norplant is the trademark for an implantable contraceptive capsule. 99395 Periodic comprehensive preventive medicine reevaluation and management. Report both.

209. b. 11106-59. This question asks how to report the biopsy procedure, not the excision. Biopsies of different lesions or different sites on the same date as another procedure are reported separately. Append Modifier -59 to identify that there were two separate lesions.

210. a. 63090, 22558-51, 22585, 22845, 20931. The primary procedure is a partial corpectomy (you can find this in the CPT Professional Edition index under corpectomy). An arthrodesis was done in addition to the definitive procedure; therefore modifier -51 is necessary (you can find this in the subcategory guidelines under Arthrodesis). Do not attach modifier -51 to add-on codes (see Appendix A for this definition). You would report the code for a structural allograft.

211. a. 27236. One way to find this answer is in the index of the CPT Professional Edition under Fracture, Femur, Neck, Open Treatment. There is an illustration under the code 27236 for a prosthetic replacement.

212. a. 76. You can find this answer in the CPT Professional Edition in the main section guidelines for the Musculoskeletal System.

213. d. 20102. One way to find this answer is in the index of the CPT Professional Edition under Wound, Exploration, Back.

214. b. 27562, S83.006A, W14.XXXA , Y92.099. Refer to the index of the CPT Professional Edition under Dislocation, Patella closed treatment for a code range. It is necessary to look up the code range and read the descriptions to select the correct code. You can find the ICD-10-CM codes under Dislocation, patella, open. The E code Alphabetic listing is in Volume 2, Section 3. Look up, Fall, (from off), tree; the second code, look up Accident, (occurring at in), house.

215. c. 24138-RT. This question asks for you to report the procedure. There is not enough information to report the evaluation and management code. You can find the procedure in the index of the CPT Professional Edition under Sequestrectomy, Olecranon Process. The modifier -RT provides additional information.

216. c. 23474, keyword is humeral AND glenoid component.

217. a. 27301-50. Modifier -50 indicates a bilateral procedure. You can find this procedure in the index of the CPT Professional Edition under Incision and Drainage, Hematoma, Knee.

218. b. 22526, 22527, 77021-26. Find In the index of the CPT Professional Edition under Annuloplasty. 77002 cannot be reported with the 22526/7. The professional service requires the reporting of modifier -26.

219. d. 51. You can find codes exempt from modifier -51 in Appendix E of the CPT Professional Edition. You could also look up each code and locate the symbol that indicates modifier -51 exempt.

220. b. 27043-RT. Right hip, subcutaneous and soft tissue.

221. b. Code 39000 is a cervical approach, code 39010 reports a transthoracic approach.

222. a. 30450. This is a secondary rhinoplasty with major revision. The closure is bundled with the surgical procedure. Modifier -78 isn't required because the second service was not performed within the postoperative period. Generally, the maximum postoperative period is no more than 90 days.

223. d. 32654. A surgical thoracoscopy always includes a diagnostic thoracoscopy. You can find this note in the CPT Professional Edition under the Thoracoscopy heading.

224. c. 33512, 33530, 35572. The code 33530 and 35572 are add-on codes and should not have modifier -51 appended. Review modifier -51 in Appendix A of the CPT Professional Edition for this note.

225. a. Placement of all distal extensions, if required. You can find this under the heading of Endovascular Repair of Descending Thoracic Aorta in the CPT Professional Edition. Read the guidelines before the section carefully and you will see the primary codes listed with find “include placement of all distal extensions”. The code description reads “plus descending thoracic aortic extensions.”

226. a. The code 33210 reports a temporary transvenous single chamber pacemaker. There is not enough information in the question to code for the placement of the permanent system.

227. d. 33235, 33217-51. When coding for this procedure, it is necessary to code for the removal (33235) and then replacement of the leads (33217). Modifier -51 indicates multiple procedures in the same anatomic site.

228. b. The code 36592 describes this procedure. You can find this answer in the index of the CPT Professional Edition under Collection and Processing, Specimen, Venous Catheter.

229. b. The code 37186 is an add-on code and would be reported in addition to the primary procedure. The guidelines preceding this procedure clearly state, do not report 37184–37185 with code 37186.

230. b. Z12.11, D12.6, Z80.0, 45384. Z12.11, Encounter for screening for malignant neoplasm of colon. D12.6, Benign neoplasm of colon, unspecified. Z80.0, Family history of malignant neoplasm of digestive organs. 45384, Colonoscopy, flexible; with removal of tumor (s), polyp(s), or other lesions by hot biopsy forceps. This answer must have the diagnosis codes and procedure code. The diagnoses codes report special screening for the colonoscopy, family history of colon cancer, and benign polyps of the colon. The procedure code 45384 reports a therapeutic procedure with removal of the polyps.

231. d. 49900. You can find this answer in the index of the CPT Professional Edition under Suture, Abdomen.

232. d. 40843. You can find this answer in the index of the CPT Professional Edition under Vestibuloplasty. You can find the definition of the vestibule of the mouth at the beginning of the digestive system above code 40800. Modifier -50 isn't necessary because the code description states "bilateral."

233. a. 41019, 77002-26. You should append modifier -26 to the radiology code to indicate the professional portion of this procedure. You can find this procedure in the index of the CPT Professional Edition under Placement, Needle, Interstitial Radioelement Application, Head.

234. c. 49450, 99152, 99153. This is a replacement procedure via the same access site. The same provider who does the procedure reports the moderate sedation codes. You can find the rules for moderate sedation in Appendix G of the CPT Professional Edition.

235. a. 49616, 11005-51, 49594. Modifier -51 is not attached to add on codes (see Appendix A).

236. c. The code 45320 includes moderate sedation.

237. a. 43274. Endoscopic retrograde cholangiopancreatography (ERCP); with placement of endoscopic stent into biliary or pancreatic duct, including pre- and post-dilation and guide wire passage, when performed, including sphincterotomy, when performed, each stent.

238. c. 99283, 49084, 74018. 49084 - Peritoneal lavage, including imaging guidance, when performed. Peritoneal lavage is a test used to determine the presence or absence of internal bleeding within the abdomen. Injury to the abdomen can result from blunt forces (i.e. motor vehicle accidents) and from penetrating objects (knife wounds and bullets). 49329 Unlisted laparoscopy procedure. ER visit is a 99283 per CPT and 74018 is same for all so not a factor.

239.c. 47563. Always review how the procedure is being performed – laparoscopy, excision, etc. This is a key to finding and reporting the correct code.

240. c. 50380, 50240-51. The code 50380 reports the auto-transplantation and reimplantation of a kidney. The parenthetical note under this code directs the use of the code for nephrectomy with modifier -51.

241. b. 55875, 77778. The code 55875 represents the procedure and the code 77778 is the clinical brachytherapy. Code 77778 includes admission to the hospital and daily visits. You can find this rule in the subcategory guidelines for Clinical Brachytherapy in the CPT Professional Edition.

242. a. 50590. This is a lithotripsy, extracorporeal shock wave treatment. You can find this procedure in the index of the CPT Professional Edition under Lithotripsy.

243. d. 54830. You can find this answer in the CPT Professional Edition index under Excision, Lesion, Epididymis. Be careful with the index in this section and follow it to lesion or you may use the incorrect code.

244. a. 54440-79. You can find this procedure in the index of the CPT Professional Edition under Repair, Penis, Injury. You would report modifier -79 for the unrelated procedure during a post-operative period by the same physician.

245. b. The code 58671 reports this procedure via a laparoscopic approach. Modifier -50 is not necessary to report a bilateral procedure due to the code description of oviducts (which is bilateral).

246. c. The code 50385 includes the conscious sedation, radiological supervision, and interpretation. The code defines a removal and replacement so there is one code to describe the entire procedure.

247. d. The code 51785 describes this procedure. The guidelines under urodynamics indicate…"When the physician only interprets the results and/or operates the equipment, a professional component, modifier -26, should be used to identify physicians' services."

248. b. You can find this code in the index of the CPT Professional Edition under Prostate, Enucleation. The vasectomy procedure is bundled with code 52649.

249. d. 59610 - 59622. You can find this information in the CPT Professional Edition under the Delivery After Previous Cesarean Delivery subsection.

250. d. None of the answers are correct. 57283 Colpopexy, vaginal; intra-peritoneal approach (uterosacral, levator myorrhaphy). See the list of codes that cannot be reported with this code in the CPT manual. Do not to report the following codes: 57556, 58263, 58270, 58280, 58292, and 58294, with code 57283, since those codes already include enterocele repair.

251. a. 67229 -50. The note under Prophylaxis indicate that these services are repetitive, performed in multiple sessions, and are intended to include all services in a defined treatment period. The parenthetical note under code 67229 states to use modifier -50 for a bilateral procedure. The operating microscope is bundled into this procedure. Refer to code 69990 for a list of bundled codes.

252. d. 69970. One way to answer this question is to look in the index of the CPT Professional Edition under the main heading of Tumor.

253. b. 60300 x 2, 77012-26. The professional services for the CT should have a modifier -26. The professional service is the procedure; therefore, there would be no modifier - 26 on code 60300.

254. a. 61001. This question represents a subsequent tap. The code 61000 is reported for an initial procedure. Modifier -50 is not necessary because it is inherently included in the code description.

255. b. 69949-50. The original code 69840 was deleted in 2018 due to low usage. You can now use 69949 for this procedure. You would attach modifier - 50 to indicate a bilateral procedure.

256. c. 61606. Each surgeon should report the work he or she completed. Because Dr. Martin completed the definitive procedure, use code 61606, which includes the repair and graft.

257. d. The code 63050 reports two or more vertebral segments, therefore, there is no need to change the units. You could find this answer by looking in the index of the CPT Professional Edition under Laminoplasty.

258. a. The decompression or freeing of intact nerve from scar tissue, including external neurolysis and/or transposition. You can find this answer in the Tabular List under Neuroplasty. You may have to look up Neuroplasty in the index first (multiple codes) and then go to the Tabular List.

259. c. 64857, 64859, 64876. Code 64857 describes suturing of a major peripheral nerve in the leg without transposition. The add-on code 64859 is used for the second major peripheral nerve. The add-on code 64876 reports the shortening of the bone. Add-on codes should not have modifier -51 attached (see Appendix A).

260. a. The code 65273 is reported for hospitalization. The code 65272 is for without hospitalization.

261. b. A new patient is one who has not received any professional services from the physician or another physician of the exact same specialty and subspecialty who belongs to the same group practice, within the past three years. You can find this answer in the E & M Guidelines and on the Decision Tree for New vs. Established Patients (same guidelines) in the CPT Professional Edition.

262. d. 99403. Counseling and/or risk factor reduction intervention services are provided to patients with symptoms or established illness.

263. a. 99291, 99292. The guidelines for critical care have a list of services that are included with critical care when performed by the physician providing the critical care and these services should not be reported separately.

264. c. 99214. This is an established patient visit and meets two of the three key components for a 99214 level visit.

265. b. 99222. The subcategory guidelines for Initial Hospital Care state, "When the patient is admitted to the hospital as an inpatient in the course of an encounter in another site of service (e.g., hospital, emergency department, observation status in a hospital, physician's office, nursing facility) all evaluation and management services provided by that physician in conjunction with that admission are considered part of the initial hospital care when performed on the same date as the admission. Therefore, the services are reported with the initial hospital care code only. The office visit is a bundled service.

266. d. None of the answers are correct. These services are all included. Exceptions and Inclusions in the guidelines should be highlighted or added to the margins for quick reference.

267. a. 93793. This question deals with outpatient anticoagulant management. The code 93793 gives specific parameters for reporting.

268. d. 99223, 99232, 99232, 99231, 99239. Day one admission or initial hospital care is 99223. Days two and three are subsequent hospital care services at 99232 and you should report them separately. Day four is subsequent hospital care at level 99231. Day five is the discharge service, which is based on time and code 99239 is reported for services of more than 30 minutes, regardless of the actual time. Report this code only once.

269. d. 99291, 99292 x 2; for 120 minutes. 99184 combines total and selective hypothermia in a critically ill neonate per day (List separately in addition to code for primary procedure and can only be reported once per hospital stay. 99184 replaces 99481 and 99482 and moved from EM to Medicine). Quantity is 2 days.

270. b. 99205. This is a new patient visit not a consultation. "A "consultation" initiated by a patient and/or family, and not requested by a physician or other appropriate source, is not reported using the consultation codes but may be reported using the office visit, home service, or domiciliary/rest home care codes." Report a consultation code only when a request (written or verbal) is made by another physician or appropriate source, an opinion is rendered, and a written report is sent back to the "requestor." In this case the patient initiated the visit.

271. a. 99485. You can find this definition in the CPT Professional Edition under the subcategory guidelines for Emergency Department Services.

272. d. 99382. Preventive medicine services are based on new vs. established patient and age.

273. b. 00832-P2, 99100. You should report the anesthesia services with modifier -P2 for mild systemic disease and qualifying circumstances due to the patient's age.

274. c. 93315. Refer to Appendix G in the CPT Professional Edition. This appendix lists the codes that include moderate conscious sedation along with guidelines to assist with reporting these services. Additionally, code 93315 has a "bulls-eye" symbol that indicates moderate conscious sedation is included with the service.

275. d. 00142-P3, 99100. According to the Anesthesia Guidelines in the CPT Professional Edition, the preoperative visit is "bundled" or included in the anesthesia services.

276. b. 43305-47. According to the Anesthesia Guidelines in the CPT Professional Edition, "To report regional or general anesthesia provided by a physician also performing the services for which the anesthesia is being provided, see modifier -47 in Appendix A." Appendix A describes the use of modifier -47 for a basic service when the anesthesia is provided by the surgeon.

277. a. Swan-Ganz monitoring. 99485. On E & M codes be sure to circle and highlight location, type (critically ill, pediatric) limiting phrases (before transport) and time.

278. c. 23. You can find the definition for Modifier -23 – Unusual Anesthesia in Appendix A of the CPT Professional Edition.

279. a. 77067-26. Screening mammography, bilateral (2-view study of each breast), including computer-aided detection (CAD) when performed.

280. c. The code 76942 is the correct code to report this procedure According to the CPT Assistant, Apr 05:15-16, “From a CPT coding perspective, code 76942 should be reported per distinct lesion that requires separate needle placement. Therefore, if passes are made into two separate lesions in the same organ (i.e., two lesions in same breast), then code 76942 would be reported twice.”

281. b. 77080-26. You can find this study in the index of the CPT Professional Edition under DXA (with a cross reference). This study was completed on the axial skeleton.

282. d. Creatinine is not part of a liver panel

283. c. Knees and small joints of the hands and feet

284. d. Parkinson disease

285. b. Herniorrhaphy

286. d. Prothrombin time

287. b. Myelominingocele

288. d. Limbic system

289. a. 69620, Myringoplasty (surgery confined to drumhead and donor area).

290. d. 69635, Tympanoplasty with antrotomy or mastoidotomy (including canalplasty, atticotomy, middle ear surgery, and/or tympanic membrane repair); without ossicular chain reconstruction.

291. a. OB. Genetic Testing Modifiers are listed in Appendix I of the CPT Professional Edition. The note under the subcategory Cytogenetic Studies refers to Appendix I.

292. a. 82075. The math calculations are included (bundled) with chemistry tests. You can find this note in the last paragraph under the Chemistry subsection of the CPT Professional Edition.

293. a. The code 80505 reports a pathology clinical consultation; for a highly complex clinical problem, with comprehensive review of patient's history and medical records and high level of medical decision making. When using time for code selection, 41-60 minutes of total time is spent on the date of the consultation. The patient was not present; therefore you would not report an evaluation and management consultation code.

294. c. 81007. You can find this answer by looking in the index of the CPT Professional Edition under Urinalysis, Semiquantitative. The bacteriuria screen, is for the infectious agent.

295. a. Lipid panel results including total cholesterol, HDL-C, triglycerides, calculated LDL-C. You can find this code in Category II codes.

296. d. The code 82272 states, "…performed for other than colorectal neoplasm screening."

297. c. 83993. You can find this test in the CPT Professional Edition under Calprotectin, fecal.

298. a. 92557-52. The description under code 92557 lists the codes that are combined and should not be reported separately. In addition, the subcategory guidelines for the Audiologic Function Tests with Medical Diagnostic Evaluation state to add modifier -52 if studies are completed on one ear.

299. b. 90471, 90472 x 2, 90717, 90746, 90691. Administration of vaccines are reported according to the route and the age of the patient. These vaccines, all injections, were given to an adult patient; therefore, you would report the codes 90471 and 90472 x 2. The vaccines are reported for each type given or injected. According to the guidelines under the Vaccines, Toxoids subsection, do not report modifier -51 for the vaccines when performed with the administration procedures.

300. c. Use code 96360 to report hydration of 31 minutes to one hour.

CPT Coding Tips

Coding Tip 1:

Always read carefully the notes under the codes in the CPT™ manual. Some of these notes define terms, such as simple, intermediate, and complex wound repair. Others provide specific coding instructions applicable to specific codes.

Coding Tip 2:

Many clinicians may not consider a biopsy a therapeutic procedure. This is where a coding definition may differ from a clinical one.

Coding Tip 3:

In actual practice, particularly with "J" codes, you will need to have a generic to trade-name cross-walk. It's unlikely they will require that knowledge for the exam except for possibly the most common generic names.

ICD-10 Coding Tips

Coding Tip 4:

We will add ICD-10 specificity to our "gray area" list. As a coder we are taught to always report the most accurate and specific codes. Often providers will argue that the level of detail in ICD-10 is unnecessary, if you treat the condition the same either way.

Coding Tip 5:

The neoplasm codes do not follow the "H" code conventions for right and left. While not common, the ICD-10 convention for right and left is a "1" for right and a "2" for left. Observe these neoplasm codes.

Coding Tip 6:

Not reporting a neoplasm on the correct side could cause legal, compliance, and auditing problems. It is not a trivial issue. Sometimes ICD-10 is not consistent and can be confusing, specially to someone new to coding.

Coding Tip 7:

The "C" neoplasm codes do not follow the same coding convention of the "H" eye and ear codes. The "H" codes for mechanical entropion includes sixth-character options 1-6 and 9 to indicate which eyelid. The "C" codes use 11, 12, 21, and 22 to indicate which of the four eyelids.

Coding Tip 8:

Chemical burns are not coded as a burn, but a corrosion. Alert the front office that if a patient states that they burned their eye or hand with caustic lye, it is not documented (or coded) as a burn but a corrosion of the eye or hand. Be sure everyone asks the question, " how did you burn yourself?" The example below illustrates eye codes as an example.

HCPCS Coding Tips

Coding Tip 9:

If an appropriate HCPCS Level II code exists, it takes precedence over a CPT™ code in Medicare/Medicaid billing (remember the supplies code?). An increasing number of private insurance carriers are also encouraging or requiring the use of certain HCPCS codes.

Coding Tip 10:

What happened to Level III HCPC codes, also known as "local codes?" These alphanumeric codes used a prefix of S, W-Z, and followed by 4 numeric digits. These codes were eliminated by CMS in 2003.

Coding Tip 11:

The most common HCPCS codes used in primary care are the G (Medicare codes) and the J codes for injectables. If you work in physical therapy or orthopedics you will need to learn the "L" orthotic supply codes.

Coding Tip 12:

Always pay attention to the HCPCS "J"code dosage and multiply it accurately for the dosage given. If the HCPCS dosage is listed as 10 mg and the actual dosage is 50 mg then the units will be 5.

Coding Tip 13:

Most HCPCS codes do not have multiply quantities so you must use the appropriate quantity in the units' column.

Coding Tip 14:

HCPCS modifiers include the location codes for the fingers (Fx), Toes (Tx), Eyelids (Ex), Left (-LT) and Right (-RT). These are used with both CPT and HCPCS codes (remember that CPT™ Codes are HCPCS codes). Therefore if you excise a benign lesion from the patient's right arm and the size is 0.5 cm or less, to get paid you must report code 11400-RT for the right arm.

CPT Modifier Coding Tips

Coding Tip 15:

The CPC exam is open book but don't think that inserting 20 pages of notes and diagrams will help you. You will have precious little time to refer to any of them. You must be able to find a particular modifier or type of E & M within seconds, not minutes. So the challenge is locating information very quickly and then eliminating wrong answers.

Coding Tip 16:

You should be aware that you can use CPT modifiers on HCPCS codes. Conversely, you can use HCPCS modifiers on CPT™ codes. In other words, when billing a carrier that accepts the full HCPCS system, you can use any modifier on any code, as long as the use is appropriate.

Coding Tip 17:

Modifiers are a great way to eliminate wrong answers on an exam. If some codes have modifiers and others do not you can eliminate answers without looking up the CPT code! Learn your modifiers. They will be a great help on the actual exam.

Coding Tip 18:

Review modifiers often. Unless it's something very specific, you should not have to look them up. Grouping them, this is very important; some are ASC only, some impact reimbursement, others are information only. Some are E & M only, others are surgical only. Compare and contrast them.

Coding Tip 19:

RVU's are not in the CPT manual therefore you won't know exactly the values unless you look them up on the Medicare website, download the file, or use an RVU reimbursement book.

Coding Tip 20:

Some clinics no longer add modifier -51 and report not having any problems. With advances in computer technology it does not appear to be necessary for most carriers. It is considered accurate coding but don't be surprised if no one uses it in your office.

Coding Tip 21:

Some coders mistakenly use the "-52" modifier to reduce a charge for a patient who is indigent. The physician performed the procedure or service as described, but did not want to charge the patient the full amount. The "-52" modifier should not be used for this purpose.

Coding Tip 22:

MOD-56 (pre-op care only) is rarely (if ever) used in the actual practice. I do not know of any carrier that pays on this modifier. However, it could show up on a coding exam.

Coding Tip 23:

Major surgery is any procedure with a 90-day global. Even if it is a short, twenty minute operation, if it has a 90-day global its considered major surgery. Some providers may use a more clinical definition assuming any procedure with general anesthesia or any procedure performed in the hospital is major. This is where a coding definition would differ from commonly-accepted clinical definitions. That will happen more than once in coding.

Coding Tip 24:

Modifier 58 (Staged or Related Procedure or Service by the Same Physician During the Postoperative Period) is often confused with MOD-78, return to the operating room. There is a lot of gray area on which code would be accurate and some carriers do not agree. Ultimately the carrier's interpretation is what counts because they reimburse you!

Coding Tip 25:

You will find examples for these modifiers in the AMA Assistant Archives, the Medicare website, as well as coding forums online. The CPT definition is not very descriptive and there are numerous interpretations of what exactly "distinct" means. Welcome to medical coding!

Coding Tip 26:

If MOD-62 is allowed it's a flag in the PFSRVU database. Once again it's not a likely question on a coding exam but really important to know when working with a surgical practice.

Coding Tip 27:

A patient is brought to the hospital with internal hemorrhaging which is repaired surgically. Three days after surgery, the patient begins hemorrhaging again and the surgeon must perform the same repair again. Would you use the repeat procedure modifier on the second repair? Yes, assuming the same procedure code was being reported. If a different physician had performed the second repair, he/she would use Modifier -77. It may be necessary to send a special report with the claim explaining why the procedure needed to be repeated. This is appropriate in cases where the need for the repeat may not be clear to the carrier. If you do not use the repeat procedure modifier the submission will most likely be denied as a duplicate claim.

Coding Tip 28:

If tests are rerun to confirm initial results, or because of testing problems with the specimen or equipment, or for any other reason when the test is normally run once, DO NOT use Modifier -91. Be sure to highlight this modifier in your manual. While it is not commonly reported it is good to know.

Coding Tip 29:

Using Multiple Modifiers. Add modifier -99 if two or more different modifiers are added to the same procedure. This alerts the carrier to the fact that two or more modifiers are associated with the procedure. While this is considered accurate coding, in actual practice it's rarely used and on occasion, a "by-the-rules" coder will confuse a carrier and be asked to stop using a code!

Evaluation & Management Coding Tips

Coding Tip 30:

There are two main E & M concepts. (1) The different type of E & M codes such as office visits, critical care, hospital admissions and emergency room visits. (2). The level and selection of a specific code: This is based on whether the patient is new or established and the level of services provided during the visit. Some codes are selected by the age of the patient.

Coding Tip 31:

Create index cards for every category or type of E & M code. You can also create cards for the number of HPI components (8), the comprehensive exam (18) and the ROS list (14).

Coding Tip 32:

Learn the Code Groups. These are in the CPT™ manual under Evaluation and Management (e.g., 99202, 99219, etc). Learn the components of E & M (History, Exam, MDM). These are in the blue guidelines section preceding the E & M code section. These documents are easily found online. Medicare 1995 E & M Guidelines. Medicare 1997 E & M Guidelines.

Coding Tip 33:

Create a set of index cards of every E & M category and all CPT modifiers and review them every day whenever possible. Whatever it takes for you to become with familiar with the E & M categories and modifiers.

Coding Tip 34:

While home visits (99341-99350) are rare, you must know how to code these. There are five levels for a new patient and four for an established. Other than the different POS code, the requirements are the same as an office visit.

Coding Tip 35:

Medicare does not pay on Prolonged Services (not face-to-face): 99358-99359 codes. A few private carriers pay but expect 80% or more of the carriers to deny the prolonged service codes. Remember that just because it is an accurate or correct code does not guarantee payment.

Coding Tip 36:

Checkup or F/U (only) is not a Chief Complaint (CC) and must be reported as a Well Exam; The CC and history of present illness (HPI) should always reference the disease, condition, or medical reason the patient is returning, not a lab or test or medication refill. Always answer "Checkup or follow-up for what condition and how long has it been" in your Chief Complaint! Also, if there is no “presenting problem” it is a preventive visit (aka routine wellness exam).

Coding Tip 37:

Do not use the word "non-contributory" in the ROS or anywhere in the medical record. Many providers learn this clinical terminology. This term is vague and infers that the system was not reviewed and therefore cannot be counted as negative.

Coding Tip 38:

Avoid a notation: "all other systems negative" or "Review of Systems negative" for a comprehensive history. This is not allowed per the Medicare 1997 Guidelines.

Coding Tip 39:

Problem List: Many EMR systems include a problem list. This is located in the history section and includes all historical diseases and conditions. It should not be used as a substitute for your assessment or impression which is used for scoring the medical decision making for today’s visit. The MDM should only include what was managed and relevant today.

Coding Tip 40:

Do not document a comprehensive history and exam and submit the visit as over 50% counseling time. It is totally unnecessary, and looks suspicious to an auditor.

Anesthesia Coding Tips

Coding Tip 41:

Anesthesia coding and reporting is very different from other specialties. It requires learning very specific rules and guidelines that only apply to anesthesiology. A veteran 20 year coder from OB/GYN would not have a clue how to report anesthesia services without considerable training. Pay careful attention to the guidelines and modifiers. Focus on the basics realizing that it would take a significant amount of additional time to master anesthesia coding.

Coding Tip 42:

CPT guidelines state that reporting anesthesia services is appropriate when the service is performed by or under the responsible supervision of a physician.

Coding Tip 43:

Never code metacarpal and digital nerve blocks separately. They are included in the surgical package.

Coding Tip 44:

Some carriers may prefer anesthesia billed as time (minutes).

Coding Tip 45:

Four codes have been identified in CPT to qualify anesthesia procedures or services. More than one of these codes may be reported and they must be assigned along with the anesthesia codes: 99100, 99116, 99135, 99140. These codes are used only with anesthesia codes and should never be used alone. Be sure to locate and highlight them in your manual.

Coding Tip 46:

When multiple surgical procedures are performed during a single anesthetic administration, the basic value is that of the procedure with the highest unit value.

Integumentary Coding Tips

Coding Tip 47:

If, because of the patient's condition, a procedure is unusually complicated, the physician should indicate this in the documentation and the coder should append modifier -22 to the procedure code. Most carriers pay on this modifier but may require you submit documentation to support it.

Coding Tip 48:

The deeper and more complex a wound is, the higher the reimbursement. The coder becomes a valued member of the reimbursement team when they can show the clinic how to increase revenue **compliantly** with accurate documentation and reporting. Read carefully all notes for any missing services (codes).

Coding Tip 49:

For debridement, use code 11000 for the first 10%, then 11001 as needed for each subsequent 10%. Do not use modifier -51 because 11001 is an Add-On code and exempt from modifier -51.

Coding Tip 50:

The treatment of the open fractures is reported in addition to the debridement code.

Coding Tip 51:

If multiple biopsies are performed, each lesion should be coded separately. Do not use a biopsy code if the lesion was removed in its entirety. A lesion excision code (benign) or (malignant) should be reported instead of a biopsy code. The biopsy codes include simple closure.

Coding Tip 52:

When multiple wounds are repaired, add together the lengths of the wounds sharing the same site grouping and classification (simple, intermediate, or complex) and assign a single code to the repair. If more than one classification of wounds is repaired, list the more complicated as the primary procedure.

Coding Tip 53:

If a wound is closed with butterfly bandages or adhesive steri-strips, do not use repair codes. This service should be reported by utilizing an appropriate Evaluation and Management code.

Coding Tip 54:

Codes that state "with flap closure" or "with skin flap closure" include those procedures and they are not coded separately.

Coding Tip 55:

When a free skin graft is used to close a pressure ulcer or the donor site of any flap for a pressure ulcer, report the free skin graft as a separate procedure.

Coding Tip 56:

Burns are coded by location, depth, degree, and in some cases, by agent.

Coding Tip 57:

ICD-10 burn codes classify burns according to extent of body surface involved.

Coding Tip 58:

The "Rule of Nines" means that the total body surface is divided into nine percent or multiples of nine percent. An infant or child deviates from an adult because of the large surface of the child's head (adult = 9%; infant = 18%; also legs are 14% not 18%)

Description	Adult	Infant
Head	9%	18%
Arms	9% X 2	9% X 2
Trunk	18% front 18% back	18% front 18% back
Legs	18% X 2	14% X 2

Musculoskeletal Coding Tips

Coding Tip 59:

The musculoskeletal system is organized by body site with subheadings including incision, excision, repair and reconstruction, fracture/dislocation, and arthrodesis. The headings are body sites, neck, spine, humerus, elbow, etc. The subheading is the Category of Procedures. Guidelines for each subheading are consistent from one body site to another within the Musculoskeletal system. Arthroscopy codes for all sites are at the end of the Musculoskeletal Section in CPT.

Coding Tip 60:

If you are not familiar with the differences between fractures, dislocations, and sprains, be sure to spend some time getting familiar as this will help in this section.

Coding Tip 61:

If a wound does not require enlargement or the extension of dissection, Simple, Intermediate, or Complex repair codes should be utilized.

Coding Tip 62:

Most fracture care codes have a global period of 90 days except for a few specific complicated surgeries requiring a longer recovery period.

Coding Tip 63:

The type of fracture (open, compound, closed) does not have any coding correlation with the type of treatment (closed, open, or percutaneous) provided.

Coding Tip 64:

The following questions must be answered prior to coding the treatment of fractures:

1. What is the site of the fracture?
2. Is the fracture open or closed?
3. Is the fracture treatment open or closed?
4. Is the manipulation part of the treatment?
5. Is an internal or external skeletal fixation device utilized?

Coding Tip 65:

The following questions must be answered prior to coding treatment of dislocations:

1. What is the site of the dislocation?
2. Is the treatment open or closed?
3. Is the manipulation part of the treatment?
4. Does the procedure include internal or external fixation of the dislocation?

Coding Tip 66:

When you bill for applying a cast or strapping, the removal of the cast or strapping is included in your charge for the application.

Coding Tip 67:

A diagnostic arthroscopy is always included in a surgical arthroscopy. Do not bill for the diagnostic arthroscopy if both are performed at the same operative session. Report only the surgical arthroscopy to the appropriate site and make the code selection. If a biopsy of the synovial tissue is performed, it is included with the diagnostic code.

Coding Tip 68:

Cruciate Ligament Repair/ Augmentation or Reconstruction procedure may be performed when a ligament is severely damaged, torn, or unable to be repaired. In this case, the ligament is replaced with a graft of sufficient strength to restore stability to the knee. Both codes 29888 and 29889 are "arthroscopically aided."

Coding Tip 69:

More than one arthroscopy code may be reported when procedures are performed in separate compartments of the knee. For example, a patient may have a lateral meniscectomy and debridement of articular cartilage performed at the same session but in different compartments.

Coding Tip 70:

Graft codes are modifier -51 exempt.

Respiratory Coding Tips

Coding Tip 71:

The Respiratory system will be used by both ENT (ear, nose, and throat) doctors and pulmonologists, two very distinct specialties. Be sure to note the difference.

Coding Tip 72:

When an excision of nasal polyp(s) is performed on both sides of the nose, report the procedure performed on the second side by adding the bilateral modifier, -50, (or add MOD-RT and MOD-LT depending on the payer) to the code for the second side.

Coding Tip 73:

To appropriately code nasal/sinus endoscopic surgery, it is important to distinguish between the endoscopic approach/method and the intranasal approach/method when coding nasal/sinus procedures because either method can be used to accomplish the same end result or procedure.

Coding Tip 74:

When coding nasal/sinus surgery, review the operative report to determine whether the procedure was performed with or without an endoscope.

Coding Tip 75:

A diagnostic sinus endoscopy and a sinusotomy are always included in a surgical sinus endoscopy. Therefore, the diagnostic sinus endoscopy and sinusotomy are not coded and billed separately.

Coding Tip 76:

Unless otherwise stated in a procedure description, the endoscopy codes in this section are unilateral (performed on one side of the nose/nasal cavity). To report bilateral procedures, add the -50 modifier to the appropriate code.

Coding Tip 77:

The best coders uncover incorrect or missed documentation and/or reporting. They also train staff and providers how to improve documentation for office visits, surgical procedures and ICD-10 diagnosis coding.

Coding Tip 78:

When coding for a laryngoscopy, the following information must be obtained:

1. Is the procedure direct or indirect? Direct viewing: the larynx directly (direct visualization) through an instrument. Indirect viewing: the larynx by looking at its reflection in a laryngeal mirror.

2. Is the procedure diagnostic or operative? Operative means that the procedure is performed under general anesthesia.

3. Was a flexible fiber optic scope used or was it rigid?

4. What other procedures were performed (i.e., biopsy), if any, along with the endoscopy?

Coding Tip 79:

When multiple procedures are performed through the bronchial endoscope, separate codes should be reported for each procedure, when appropriate. The multiple procedure modifier -51 should be used for each subsequent procedure performed through the scope.

Coding Tip 80:

When a diagnostic thoracoscopy is immediately followed by an open thoracotomy or other open chest procedure, report both procedures. List the appropriate code for the open chest procedure first and the thoracoscopy second.

Cardiovascular Coding Tips

Coding Tip 81:

Note the distinction between cardiovascular surgery and cardiology (Medicine Section codes). The cardiovascular section starts with code 33016 and ends with 39599.

Coding Tip 82:

There is a big difference between a cardiologist and a cardiovascular or cardiothoracic surgeon. The cardiologist performs numerous tests, most found in the Medicine section, and mildly invasive therapeutic procedures such and angioplasties (also found in the Medicine section). The cardiovascular surgeon performs the heart valve replacements and bypass grafts (where you open the patient's chest).

Coding Tip 83:

A complete service, as defined by CMS, is one in which the physician provides the entire service, including equipment, supplies, technical personnel, and the physician's personal professional services. The complete service can also be divided into a technical and a professional component.

Coding Tip 84:

ECG And EKG mean the same exact thing: electrocardiogram. In CPT the acronym ECG is used in the CPT code descriptions. In actual practice you may see EKG more often.

Coding Tip 85:

In the office where the complete service is generally provided (i.e., the physician owns the equipment and employs the personnel), the physician should use the CPT code 93000 without any modifiers.

Coding Tip 86:

Exercise stress tests are commonly reported by cardiologists and some primary care providers. Codes 93015 through 93018 are used to report cardiovascular stress tests.

Coding Tip 87:

Stress testing may be performed to symptom-limited endpoints, or to a submaximal endpoint. Heart rate, blood pressure, and the electrocardiogram are monitored during the stress testing, with recording of 12-lead electrocardiographic tracings before, during, and after stress testing. If imaging modalities are used, the imaging procedures are coded separately.

Coding Tip 88:

Catheter placement codes with injection(s), imaging supervision, and interpretation 93451 - 93461. These codes describe the insertion of catheters into the various chambers of the heart or arteries, veins, and great vessels. They cover the introduction, positioning, and repositioning of the catheters, as well as recording of intracardiac and intravascular pressures, and obtaining blood samples to measure blood gases and/or dye or other dilution curves and cardiac output. These codes also include a final evaluation and report of the catheterization procedure.

Coding Tip 89:

Injection procedures for angiography performed in conjunction with cardiac catheterization and are coded in addition to the appropriate catheter placement code(s). Each code in this series may be reported only once per cardiac catheterization service.

Coding Tip 90:

When coding venous and arterial-venous grafting procedures, do not code the procurement of the saphenous vein graft separately. It is included in these codes.

Coding Tip 91:

Replacement of a battery or pulse generator for either a pacemaker or defibrillator system requires the use of two codes. One code for the removal of the pulse generator and another for the insertion of a new one.

Digestive Coding Tips

Coding Tip 92:

The digestive system set of CPT Codes has more unique medical terminology than any other section of CPT. There are over 100 terms most coders won't know without specific study.

Coding Tip 93:

If you don't know what a word means or where the organ is, it's crucial that you look it up. Some of the words are quite long and intimidating. However, if you break medical procedures down into prefixes and suffixes they are more manageable.

Coding Tip 94:

A lot of digestive system surgery involves radiological supervision and interpretation. Be sure to read the op report carefully and review the notes in parentheses under the CPT™ code and description to determine the correct radiological code.

Coding Tip 95:

Do not confuse an approach such as abdominal with a technique such as cryosurgery, fulguration, or excision. While it could be argued whether an arthroscopic procedure versus an open procedure is an approach or technique, the key here is to always find, note, and highlight both approaches and techniques and always be on the lookout for them in the surgical op report. Sometimes the provider will report the wrong code and the reimbursement can be significantly different.

Coding Tip 96:

Tonsillectomies and adenoidectomies CPT™ Codes are age-dependent. Be sure to note whether the patient is under or over age 12.

Coding Tip 97:

If a balloon catheter is used to remove the foreign body from the colon, radiological supervision and interpretation may be required. Report code 74235 in addition to code 43215 in these instances.

Coding Tip 98:

Codes 43216 and 43217 are only reported once regardless of the number of lesions treated.

Coding Tip 99:

Report code 43220 for balloon dilation less than 30 mm in diameter. If an upper gastrointestinal endoscopy is performed instead of an esophagoscopy, use CPT Code 43249 to report it.

Coding Tip 100:

All EGD codes are in the 43235 – 43259 range. Be sure to bracket or highlight these in your CPT™ manual.

Coding Tip 101:

Code 43264 is used to report the removal of stones from biliary and/or pancreatic ducts with endoscopic retrograde (ERCP). When this procedure is performed, it may be preceded by a sphincterotomy/papillotomy (43262). When both procedures are performed, report each procedure separately, listing the appropriate code for each.

Coding Tip 102:

Per instructions in the CPT manual, use modifier -53 to report an incomplete colonoscopy.

Coding Tip 103:

For a single tumor, polyp, or lesion removed by the snare technique, use code 45309. If multiple tumors, polyps or lesions are removed by hot biopsy forceps, bipolar cautery, or snare technique use code 45315.

Coding Tip 104:

If single or multiple tumors, polyps, or lesions are removed by laser, use code 45320.

Urinary System Coding Tips

Coding Tip 105:

Always read the complete text of each code and its descriptor before selecting the code. Know male and female anatomy. Learn the different complex surgical procedures.

Coding Tip 106:

A nephrostomy or pyelostomy may be done alone, without a nephrostolithotomy. To code a nephrostomy only, use code 50040, nephrostomy, nephrotomy with drainage. Use code 50045 for a Nephrotomy, with exploration. Use code 52334 for a retrograde percutaneous nephrostomy.

Coding Tip 107:

For removal or manipulation of calculi in the ureter through an endoscope, see the codes referenced in the third note below code 50630 in your CPT book.

Coding Tip 108:

Under the heading of Endoscopy: Cystoscopy, Urethroscopy, and Cystourethroscopy, there are endoscopic procedures listed from code 52000 through code 52700. These often include minor functions that are related to the main procedure and are usually considered an integral part of the main procedure. When one of these minor functions or procedures requires significant additional time and effort (for example, morbid obesity), you may append modifier -22.

Urinary System/ Female Coding Tips

Coding Tip 109:

Code 57500: Biopsy, single or multiple, or local excision of lesion, with or without fulguration (separate procedure). When a dilation and curettage is also performed, include both codes on the claim with the D & C (58120) first.

Coding Tip 110:

Code 58100: Endometrial and/or endocervical sampling (biopsy), without cervical dilation, any method (separate procedure). This code is both a separate and a starred procedure. As a separate procedure, it is usually a component of a larger surgical service and should not be billed in addition to that larger service. However, if it is performed alone, as a starred procedure, any other service (office visit or unrelated procedure) can also be billed.

Coding Tip 111:

A routine dilation and curettage before a hysterectomy should not be reported separately.

Coding Tip 112:

If an IUD is removed and another IUD inserted at the same time only the insertion code should be reported.

Coding Tip 113:

Multiple biopsies of a single mass are coded as a single procedure.

Coding Tip 114:

A diagnostic laparoscopy should not be coded separately unless it is the only procedure performed.

Coding Tip 115:

Code 58555: Hysteroscopy, diagnostic (separate procedure). This procedure is automatically included in all of the hysteroscopy codes. Do not code a diagnostic hysteroscopy separately unless it is the only procedure completed.

Coding Tip 116:

Procedures under an endoscopy subheading are not considered "open" surgical procedures.

Coding Tip 117:

A diagnostic laparoscopy is always included in a surgical laparoscopy. Therefore, when a diagnostic laparoscopy and a surgical laparoscopy are performed during the same operative session, report the surgical laparoscopy only.

Coding Tip 118:

A hysteroscopy is often accompanied by diagnostic laparoscopy to determine whether the exterior configuration of the uterus is normal or is indented in the shape of a Y (bicornate uterus). It is usually done after a vaginal ultrasound or an X-ray (hysterosalpingogram) that indicates a Y-shaped abnormality of the uterus. Because the X-ray does not show whether the distinctive shape is due to a septum within the uterus or to a uterus that is itself Y-shaped, the laparoscopy is performed first. If done, code and report both the laparoscopy and the hysteroscopy that follows.

Coding Tip 119:

Code 58260 includes only a hysterectomy and should not be reported when the tubes and ovaries are also removed.

Coding Tip 120:

The AMA did not include the statement "with or without tubes and ovaries" in this code's description. For this reason, some insurance carriers will allow separate payment for tube and ovary removal. In this case, code 58262 would be coded using modifier -51.

Urinary System/ Male Coding Tips

Coding Tip 121:

When ultrasonic guidance is used to perform a biopsy of the prostate, refer to radiological codes 76942 for reporting the ultrasonic guidance services/procedures, if appropriate.

Coding Tip 122:

To report laparoscopic repair of bilateral inguinal hernias, add modifier -50 to the appropriate code.

Coding Tip 123:

Codes: 49570 - 49572: Repair of an epigastric hernia. These procedures may be referred to as "TAPP", TransAbdominal PrePeritoneal.

Obstetrics Coding Tips

Coding Tip 124:

Obstetricians record patient histories that note parity (the number of pregnancies a woman has carried to 20 weeks), gravidity, and the results of all pregnancies. Two shorthand systems are used to record patient histories. The GPA system notes the: Gravida, Para, Abortus. The TPAL system counts: Term births, Premature births, Abortions, Living children.

Coding Tip 125:

The services normally provided in uncomplicated maternity cases include:

1. Antepartum Care
2. Delivery
3. Postpartum Care
4. Antepartum care includes
5. Initial and subsequent history
6. Physical Exams
7. Recording of weight, blood pressures, fetal heart tones
8. Routine urinalysis
9. Monthly visits up to 28 weeks
10. Bi-weekly visits 29 -36 weeks
11. Weekly visits after 36 weeks

Any other visits or services within this time period should be coded separately. When high-risk pregnancies require more visits than described above, and more laboratory data than indicated in the preceding description, these services should be reported separately, in addition to the global code for maternity care and delivery.

Coding Tip 126:

If a patient is admitted to the hospital for observation prior to delivery and stays more than 24 hours, you should report the hospital care rendered, except the day of delivery, separately.

Endocrinological Coding Tips

Coding Tip 127:

The CPT Endocrine Section is only two pages in the CPT manual. The following organs are NOT found in the Endocrine Section of CPT (even though they may have endocrine properties).

Pancreas	Digestive	48000 - 48999
Ovaries/Oviducts	Female Genital System	58600 - 58999
Testes	Male Genital System	54500 - 54699
Pituitary		61546 - 61548, 62165
Pineal gland	No CPT procedures	

Coding Tip 128:

The parotid gland is part of the salivary gland. It has nothing to do with the carotid body.

Coding Tip 129:

The review of surgical procedures of the pituitary and pineal glands are found in the Nervous System Module of CPT.

Coding Tip 130:

The thyroid gland is a part of the endocrine (hormone) system and plays a major role in regulating the body's metabolism.

Nervous System Coding Tips

Coding Tip 131:

Neurology codes 62320 through 62327 were added in 2018. Pay careful attention to the placement: cervical, thoracic, lumbar, sacral procedure: diagnostic, therapeutic, continuous infusion placement of the semicolon with or without imaging. Read all notes underneath the group of codes.

Coding Tip 132:

The peripheral nervous system includes the 12 pairs of cranial nerves, the 31 pairs of spinal nerves, and the autonomic nervous system.

Coding Tip 133:

Codes 95805 - 95829, 95921 - 95929, and 95954 - 95962 describing EEG services, include tracing, interpretation, and report.

Coding Tip 134:

Code with MOD -26 for interpretation only.

Coding Tip 135:

Health & Behavior Assessments (from the Medicine Section): 96156 - 96171. These are straightforward. Always highlight, annotate (to the side), or circle with a red pen or pencil key words.

Eye System Coding Tips

Coding Tip 136:

As with all other surgical sections, it is recommended that you scan through the eye section to obtain a "birds' eye" view of how it is organized. This will help you find codes quickly. Read the guidelines, take notes and spend no less than sixty minutes on your overview. Spend at least twenty minutes learning the anatomy of the eye.

Coding Tip 137:

Do not use code 65130 for the insertion of an IntraOcular Lens (IOL) as a secondary procedure after cataract removal. The code pertains to the secondary implant of an eyeball, not a lens.

Coding Tip 138:

CPT differentiates between a foreign body removal and removal of implanted material in the eye. A foreign body is a splinter of wood or metal, or dirt. It is not something that was purposely put into the body.

Coding Tip 139:

Multiple notes appear in the Eye Subsection to inform the coder that procedures involving only the skin of the eyelid or orbit are assigned codes from the Integumentary System.

Coding Tip 140:

While the CPT manual has numerous cataract removal codes in actual practice the overwhelming majority use code 66984 for a normal cataract surgery and to a lesser extent, code 66982 (complex) cataract surgery.

Coding Tip 141:

If adjustable sutures are used, no matter how many sutures are placed, report code 67335 just one time. This code does not require a MOD-51. However, if adjustable sutures are placed in both eyes, it is appropriate to use MOD-50.

Auditory System Coding Tips

Coding Tip 142:

Always pay careful attention to -otomy (an incision) versus an -extomy (an excision). It is easy to confuse these when coding.

Coding Tip 143:

Report tympanostomy with ventilating tubes under general anesthesia with code 69436. If the procedure is performed bilaterally, add modifier -50 to the second procedure. Report myringotomy without insertion of ventilating tubes with codes 69420 or 69421.

Coding Tip 144:

Patients with identified hearing loss receive follow-up services to monitor audiologic status and to ensure appropriate treatment. Documentation addresses interpretation of test results and the type and severity of the hearing loss and associated conditions (medical diagnosis, disability, home program).

Radiology Coding Tips

Coding Tip 145:

The radiology section of CPT is divided into four subsections which are further divided by anatomy: Diagnostic, Ultrasound, Radiation Oncology, Nuclear Medicine.

Coding Tip 146:

To code radiological procedures correctly, the coder must know what was x-rayed and, in many cases, the number of views taken. The coder must also know the exact positional views taken.

Coding Tip 147:

For both CAT scans and MRI scans, you need to determine if contrast material was used. If a scan was done without contrast material, followed by contrast materials and additional scan sections, then you should report a code specifying both without and with contrast material.

Coding Tip 148:

For a CAT Scan of the maxillofacial area without contrast, followed by contrast and additional CAT scan sections, use code 70488. Do not code with and without contrast separately.

Coding Tip 149:

If the physician performs the radiology procedure (owns the equipment), reviews and interprets the x-rays, and completes a written report, he or she would use the appropriate CPT code without a modifier. When the physician only interprets the x-rays, modifier -26, professional component, should be appended to the code (does not own the equipment and the hospital or another clinic creates the image).

Coding Tip 150:

Contrast material when used in a CT of the spine is either by intrathecal or intravenous injection. For intrathecal injection, also use 61055 or 62284. IV injection of contrast material is part of the CT procedure.

Coding Tip 151:

Diagnostic Ultrasound (76506-76999). This subsection is divided by body site. The main terms "echography" and "ultrasound" are used to locate the codes in the CPT index.

Coding Tip 152:

Abdominal ultrasound codes (76700-76705) are not to be used to report a pregnancy ultrasound. The correct codes for pregnancy ultrasound can be found under the subsection pelvis, codes 76805-76816, which refers to the pregnant uterus. Read the code description and ultrasound report carefully before choosing the appropriate code.

Coding Tip 153:

Another common coding question regards the reporting of a needle biopsy of the prostate using ultrasonic guidance. In this situation, two codes are required if the physician is performing both portions of the procedure.

Coding Tip 154:

In selecting the code from radiation treatment delivery (77401-77412), coders must know the energy level of the radiation administered.

Coding Tip 155:

Diagnostic radiopharmaceuticals, or therapeutic radiopharmaceuticals,
the radioactive elements used to conduct nuclear medicine procedures are reported separately using HCPCS codes. Consult your state Medicare LCD for a complete list of HCPCS codes and allowable drugs.

Pathology & Laboratory Coding Tips

Coding Tip 156:

Coding for Path & Lab is straightforward. Focus on the guidelines, the lab panels, and the gross pathology codes. In actual practice most lab codes are provided by the equipment, testing lab, or the pathology department. The ICD-10 coding is much more difficult in Path & Lab than the CPT coding. When presented with a long list of individual labs, bracket groups of codes and then bracket key differences.

Coding Tip 157:

The pathology and laboratory section of CPT is divided into subsections. Several of the subheadings or subsections have special instructions unique to that section. Where they are indicated (e.g., panel tests) special "notes" are presented. Be sure to specifically read and highlight each subsection.

Coding Tip 158:

Guidelines that clarify how pathology and laboratory codes should be used are found at the beginning of the section and in code categories, subcategories, and parenthetical phrases throughout the section. The guidelines are in the same arrangement as the other sections of the CPT manual and are unique to the category, subcategory, range of codes, or to an individual code. List each laboratory procedure separately unless it is part of a multichannel test.

Coding Tip 159:

Modifier -51 is never used with pathology or laboratory codes.

Coding Tip 160:

Many lab tests can be performed by different methods. To choose the correct code, first determine which method was used. When in doubt, request information from the physician or laboratory for clarification, or consult an authoritative reference source.

Medicine Coding Tips

Coding Tip 161:

Most of the Medicine section information is in the specific specialty areas. For example, catheterizations are in the cardiology section and the Ophthalmological exams will be in the Eye section. Some information, like the psychology codes, will be listed here. As with all the other sections, you should first spend time reviewing and highlighting the guidelines and scanning through the section. The medicine section can be daunting. It's nearly impossible to learn and memorize every type of test for every specialty plus all the corresponding guidelines. Your goal is to know what types of tests are in the medicine section.

Coding Tip 162:

In some cases the services listed in this section may be performed in conjunction with services or procedures listed in other sections of CPT. It may be appropriate to use multiple codes from different section of CPT to identify multiple services/procedures performed.

Coding Tip 163:

Note that immunization procedure codes include the supplies and the vaccine. When an immunization is given, the administration codes (90471 - 90474) should be reported in addition to the immunization code.

Coding Tip 164:

New combination immunizations have been introduced in the past several years which combine vaccines in one injection to reduce the number of needle sticks required for the patient. An example of a combination immunization is code 90723. This immunization injection includes: Diphtheria, Tetanus toxoids, Acellular pertussis vaccine (DTaP), Hemophilus influenza B (HIB). In this case only one code (one injection) should be reported.

Coding Tip 165:

Therapeutic or Diagnostic Infusions (excludes chemotherapy). Codes listed in this subsection should be reported to describe prolonged intravenous infusion requiring the presence, or under direct supervision, of the physician. These codes are reported based on time.

Coding Tip 166:

Therapeutic or Diagnostic Injections. This subsection is used to describe subcutaneous, intramuscular, intra-arterial, and intravenous injections for diagnostic and/or therapeutic purposes. These codes should not be used for allergen immunotherapy injections.

Coding Tip 167:

Note that the code descriptor requires that the specific substance injected should be reported with an additional code (specify material injected). Again, third-party payer policies vary on the type of codes used. For Medicare, HCPCS Level II J codes, or in some cases G codes, are required. If additional services are performed at the time of an injection they should be reported separately.

Coding Tip 168:

In reporting psychotherapy, the appropriate code is chosen on the basis of the type of psychotherapy. In the past several years major changes were made to the selection of CPT new encounter codes. Most mental health professionals have to report E & M codes for their encounters and they don't match up exactly with how they were trained.

Coding Tip 169:

Use Code 90901 for all biofeedback training by any modality.

Coding Tip 170:

The Dialysis subsection describes services for End-Stage Renal Disease (ESRD), hemodialysis, peritoneal dialysis, and miscellaneous dialysis procedures. Read the guidelines and code descriptors carefully in this section.

Coding Tip 171:

When linking diagnoses to CPT™ Codes in box 24e do not link all of them to each code. (A, B, C, D, E etc). This is commonly done and is incorrect. Always link a specific ICD-10 code with the appropriate CPT code. This is directly related to reimbursement and not the actual selection of a code but linking for medical necessity.

Coding Tip 172:

Evaluation and management services related to the patient's end stage renal disease that are rendered on the same day when dialysis is performed, and all other patient care services that are rendered during the dialysis procedure, are included in the dialysis procedure. Evaluation and management services unrelated to the dialysis procedure that cannot be rendered during the dialysis session may be reported in addition to the dialysis procedure.

Coding Tip 173:

Contact lens services are not considered part of general ophthalmological services, and therefore can be reported separately. Few if any carriers will pay.

Coding Tip 174:

Evaluation and Management service codes are utilized to report diagnostic or treatment procedures usually included in a comprehensive otorhinolaryngologic evaluation or office visit. Special diagnostic and treatment services, such as laryngeal function studies or nasal function studies, which usually are not included in a comprehensive otorhinolaryngologic evaluation or office visit, are reported separately using codes from the 92500 series.

Coding Tip 175:

Hand-held Doppler devices (like those used in the emergency room department) are considered part of the vascular system physical examination, and as such are not reported separately.

Coding Tip 176:

As a coder (and biller) it is important to note that often you can bill for the administration of drugs (J Codes). Codes 96372 - 96376 are the most common. Spend a little extra time on these. For one, in Primary Care they are very common and used nearly every day. Second, they can be confusing. It is important that you organize them by type, time, and method. One method is to organize them all on a single page using boxes and colored pencils.

Coding Tip 177:

As a coder you should make the doctors aware of the different codes and their wording. They may not be aware that changing or adding a few words can make a big difference in reimbursement. This is where the coder can maximize their value to the clinic. Also the coder should review the RVU's for all the different debridement codes and create a spreadsheet so it's clear which pay the most. While not specifically a coding function, you may work with either billing or finance to create this report.

Coding Tip 178:

Many payers may not reimburse for some or all of the Special Services, Procedures and Reports codes. To avoid bill rejection or claim delays, review your payer manual before submitting these codes.

Coding Tip 179:

Codes 99050 and 99058 are used when the physician provides services during hours when the office is not normally open or on an emergency basis. While most clinics rarely report these codes, I have found that a select few insurance carriers do pay (roughly 10-15%). You could win some points in a new practice if you add these to the fee ticket and actually get paid. These codes are reported in addition to the E & M code. These codes cannot be used if the clinic is open 24 hours. Both are not reimbursed by Medicare but a few carriers, in any given city, will pay on them.

Pain Management Coding Tips

Coding Tip 180:

While pain management is most often associated with anesthesia, the CPT™ codes are mostly from the Nervous System section.

Coding Tip 181:

If you do not currently work in a medical office it's difficult to know common and even simple answers such as "how is a specific drug most often injected?" Is it IV or IM? Is it a push or infusion technique? These are not trivial questions and someone new to healthcare should spend extra time learning about the different injection types.

Coding Tip 182:

Pain management procedures that may be coded and billed as appropriate within carrier reporting and coverage guidelines include:

1. Injections into the structures surrounding the spinal cord
2. Injections into specific nerves
3. Regional IV administration of local anesthetic
4. Intravenous or intra-arterial therapy during procedures for disease related pain
5. Daily management of epidural or subarachnoid drug administration

Coding Tip 183:

There is no laboratory or imaging test to establish the diagnosis of trigger point pain. Documentation must be accurate and thorough.

Coding Tip 184:

When pain management injections are given, an epidural is generally given first. The coder should determine the number of injections given and the location of each. If the procedure is bilateral, modifier -50 should be added. If radiological guidance was utilized, it should be additionally coded.

Secrets To Reducing Exam Stress

What is Stress

Stress is a normal physical response to events that make you feel threatened or upset your balance in some way, such as situations beyond your control. The body reacts to these situations with physical, mental, and emotional responses that all merge to create what is known as stress.

Remember the first time someone reprimanded you for something you had done wrong? Not necessarily a parent or relative, but someone in school or at your place of employment where you felt threatened and began feeling stressed and nervous? That was a natural reaction to a set of circumstances that caused you to feel the effects of stress. This can be a good thing during an emergency or other event but can also be a bad thing when you are trying to concentrate or think clearly during an exam.

What Causes Stress and Anxiety

Stress is caused by fear, plain and simple. The fear of the unknown. The fear of failing. The fear of being unprepared. The fear of an uncontrollable situation. Anything beyond our control can cause fear or a sense of danger and this causes the body to release stress hormones, thus increasing your stress and anxiety level. There are other factors that cause stress too but the main focus of this book is stress directly attributed to exam preparation and taking an exam.

Once you learn how to reduce and manage stress for an exam you can certainly expand its uses to other areas of your life as well. As a matter of fact, I highly recommend that you do. The facts are clear, the less stress you have in your life the longer you will live and the better quality of life you will have.

Learn to Relax

Setting your mind at ease and learning how to relax can reduce stress dramatically. This is much easier said than done, however, there are different techniques to help you relax and each have there own set of benefits. There are many different ways to relax your mind and body. Some are more difficult than others. Let's begin with an easy way to reduce even the most sever cases of stress.

Slow Your Breathing

When you begin to feel the effects of stress your breathing accelerates and your heart rate quickens. This is caused by adrenaline being pumped into your system from the body's reaction to a circumstance or situation.

The easiest and fastest way to reduce your stress level is to slow your breathing. Give this method a try. Take a deep breath and exhale slowly. Repeat this several times until your muscles are totally relaxed and your heart rate slows. Use this method before studying and prior to and during the exam itself! It will help you think more clearly and be able to recall learned information more rapidly.

Develop Your Concentration

Concentration is described as "intense mental application; complete attention".

It is your minds ability to focus on the task at hand and block out all other influences and distractions. To concentrate on one thing and one thing exclusively... the exam.

Information Retention

Your ability to concentrate is vital to your exam success. The more you concentrate on the subject materials the better you will retain and recall the information when the time comes to perform.

For you to perform your best, all attention must be on the study material and the exam. This deep level of concentration will help you maximize your study time. In most cases, the better you can concentrate during your study time the less study time you will actually have to schedule. The saying "quality over quantity" applies to exam preparation too! **Study Smarter, Not Longer!**

Power of Positive Thinking

Positive thinking can reduce stress, improve your overall health, and make you much more interesting and fun to be around. Although it is unclear exactly why positive thinkers experience health benefits, one of the theories is it helps them deal with stressful situations better. They are thinking of the best outcome, not the worst outcome, and this creates less stress and anxiety. This is better for the mind and the body.

Optimists (or positive people) always consider the "what if it could work" side of things. They are happy and easy with a smile. They give as much positive energy as they get from others and are usually interesting and fun to be around. An optimist is more likely to be successful too. They "will their self to victory". They tell THEMSELVES they can do something and this starts the ball of positivity and success rolling.

Self Talk

Why is self talk important? Well, the mind is always thinking and creating "self-talk". Self-talk is the endless stream of thoughts that run through your head. Self-talk is based on information, reason, logic, and prior experience. Self-talk also comes from misconceptions created because of misinformation or lack of information. This can be negative or positive, depending on your outlook.

Programing your self talk will help you control the way you look at things and the attitude you have towards them. Self-talk is enormously powerful and you want to have it on your side.

Train Your Mind

In the end, the mind will do what you <u>train</u> it to do. It is our job to change the way we think. Think positive thoughts. "I CAN do this." "I <u>will</u> pass the exam." Train your mind to think positively and this will reduce your stress level and give you a confident feeling going into the exam.

Do not let others, or your surroundings, dictate your mental state of mind. <u>YOU</u> have the ultimate control and <u>YOU</u> control whether you think positive or negative thoughts.

The first "YES I CAN", and "I CAN DO WHATEVER I PUT MY MIND TO" will begin the change. It will start the little snowball rolling down the mountain... and with a little momentum comes massive change!

Developing Confidence

Confidence is developed through a series of "wins" or "achievements". It is developed through facing your fears and overcoming them. This gives you strength and confidence in your ability to overcome. The more you overcome, the more confident you become.

So how do you build confidence in your ability to pass an exam? Simple.... preparation! Face your fears head on and take action. Prepare every day until you know you are going to pass... there is not doubt!

Confidence and the Exam

Your confidence will have a direct effect on your exam results. If you are confident in your ability to pass the exam it lowers your stress level and opens your mind for clearer thinking. When you project confidence your body reacts differently to circumstances. It gives you the calmness to perform at a high level.

Sleep

Why is sleep so important? Because it is the only time your body has a chance to recharge. A good sleep regiment should consist of at least six hours of sleep each night so your body and mind are fresh and ready to go the next morning. Anything less and you will not be fully rested and your performance will suffer because of it.

What If I Fail?

The most successful people fail all the time! It is a result of taking action. There is no shame in failure, only shame in not getting back up, learning from your mistakes and trying again. Overcome your fear of failure and success will be yours. If you have prepared properly you will not fail. But if you should, embrace it, be accountable for it, and start again with more resolve than ever.

Getting Help

Is there a certain section of material that is just not making sense or sinking in? GET HELP! Don't wait or, worse yet, be too shy to ask for help. Search out help as fast as you can. Many teachers and instructors are more than willing to give you a helping hand. That is their profession and most of them generally love to help people. Take advantage of their help if you need it. REMEMBER, YOU ARE NOT IN THIS ALONE!

Common Anatomical Terminology

Anatomy terminology can seem complex and overwhelming when just starting out. Once you familiarize yourself with some of the more common terms it will make your preparation much easier. Learn and few terms each day and before you know it you will have established a good base to work from. Take time to familiarize yourself with these terms to make you a better medical coder.

Anatomy Terminology - Number	
Term	**Meaning**
mono-, uni-	one
bi	two
tri	three

Anatomy Terminology - Direction and Position	
Term	**Meaning**
ab-	away from
ad-	toward
ecto-, exo-	outside
endo-	inside
epi-	upon
anterior or ventral	at or near the front surface of the body
posterior or dorsal	at or near the real surface of the body
superior	above
inferior	below
lateral	side
distal	farthest from center
proximal	nearest to center

Anatomy Terminology - Basic Terms	
Term	**Meaning**
abdominal	abdomen
buccal	cheek
cranial	skull
digital	fingers and toes
femoral	thigh
gluteal	buttocks
hallux	great toe
inguinal	groin
lumbar	lowest part of spine
mammary	breast
nasal	nose
occipital	back of head
pectoral	breastbone
thoracic	chest
umbilical	navel
ventral	belly

Anatomy Terminology - Conditions - Prefixes	
Term	**Meaning**
ambi-	both
dys-	bad, painful, difficult
eu-	good, normal
homo-	same
iso-	equal, same
mal-	bad, poor

Anatomy Terminology - Conditions - Suffixes	
Term	**Meaning**
-algia	pain
-emia	blood
-itis	inflammation
-lysis	destruction, breakdown
-oid	like
-opathy	disease of
-pnea	breathing

Anatomy Terminology - Surgical Procedures	
Term	**Meaning**
-centesis	puncture a cavity to remove fluid
-ectomy	surgical removal or excision
-ostomy	a new permanent opening
-otomy	cutting into, incision
-opexy	surgical fixation
-oplasty	surgical repair
-otripsy	crushing or destroying

Medical Terminology Prefix, Root, and Suffixes

Being familiar with Medical Terminology prefixes, roots and suffixes are essential for a medical coder. This illustrates how roots, prefixes, and suffixes are used to denote number or size, direction, color, anatomical locations, as well as other meanings.

Medical Terminology - Prefixes and Roots Denoting Number or Size	
Term	**Meaning**
bi-	two
dipl/o	two, double
hemi-	half
hyper-	over or more than usual
hypo-	under or less than usual
iso-	equal, same
macro-	large
megal/o-	enlargement
micro-	small
mono-	one
multi-	many
nulli-	none
poly-	many
semi-	half, partial
tri-	three
uni-	one

Medical Terminology - Roots Denoting Color	
Term	**Meaning**
chlor/o	green
cyan/o	blue
erythr/o	red
leuk/o	white
melan/o	black
xanth/o	yellow

Medical Terminology - Prefixes and Roots Denoting Relative Direction	
Term	**Meaning**
per-	through
peri-	around
post-	behind, after
poster/o	behind
pre-	before, in front of
pro-	before
retr/o	behind, in back of
sub-	under
super-	beyond
supra-	above
syn-	together
trans-	across
ventr/o	belly

Medical Terminology - Roots Denoting Anatomical Location	
Term	**Meaning**
abdomin/o	abdomen
acr/o	extremity
aden/o	gland
angi/o	vessel
arter/i/o	artery
arthr/o	joint
blast/o	embryo
blephar/o	eyelid
bronch/i/o	bronchus
calcane/o	calaneous
cardi/o	heart
carp/o	carpal, wrist
cephal/o	head
cerebr/o	cerebrum
cheil/o	lip
chol/e	bile, gall
chondr/o	cartilage
cocc/i	coccus
col/o	colon
colp/o	vagina
condyl/o	condyle
core/o, cor/o	pupil
corne/o	cornea

Medical Terminology - Roots Denoting Anatomical Location	
Term	**Meaning**
cost/o	ribs
crani/o	cranium
cycl/o	ciliary body
cyst/o	bladder, sac
cyt/o	cell
dactyl/o	fingers or toes
dent/o	tooth
derm/o	skin
dermat/o	skin
duoden/o	duodenum
enter/o	intestine
esophag/o	esophagus
fibr/o	fiber
gangli/o	ganglion
gastr/o	stomach
gingiv/o	gums
gloss/o	tongue
gynec/o	women
hem/o, hemat/o	blood
hepat/o	liver
hidr/o	sweat
humer/o	humerus
hydr/o	water

Medical Terminology - Roots Denoting Anatomical Location	
Term	**Meaning**
hyster/o	uterus
ile/o	ileum
irid/o, ir/o	iris
ischi/o	ischium
jejun/o	jejunum
kerat/o	cornea
lacrim/o	tear
laryng/o	larynx
lip/o	fat
lith/o	stone, calculus
lumb/o	loin, lumbar area
ment/o	chin
my/o	muscle
myel/o	spinal cord, bone marrow
nas/o	nose
nephr/o	kidney
neur/o	nerve
omphal/o	umbilicus, navel
onych/o	nail
oophor/o	ovary
opthalm/o	eye
orchid/o	testicles
oste/o	bone

Medical Terminology - Roots Denoting Anatomical Location	
Term	**Meaning**
ot/o	ear
pancreat/o	pancreas
pely/i	pelvis
peps/o/ia	digestion
phalang/o	phalange
pharyng/o	pharynx
phas/o	speech
phleb/o	veins
pleur/o	pleura
pne/o	air, breathing
pneum/o, pneumono	lung
pod/o	foot
proct/o	rectum, anus
psych/o	mind
pub/o	pubis
py/o	pus
pyel/o	kidney
rect/o	rectum
ren/o	kidney
retin/o	retina
rhin/o	nose
salping/o	fallopian tube
scler/o	sclera

Medical Terminology - Roots Denoting Anatomical Location	
Term	**Meaning**
spermat/o	sperm
splen/o	spleen
stern/o	sternum, breastbone
stomat/o	mouth
thorac/o	thorax, chest
trache/o	trachea
traumat/o	tramua
tympan/o	eardrum
ur/o	urine
ureter/o	ureter
urethr/o	urethra
vas/o	vessel
viscer/o	gut, contents of the abdomen

Medical Terminology - Other Prefixes	
Term	**Meaning**
a-, an-	without
anti-	against
auto-	self
brady-	slow
con-	with
contra-	against
dis-	free of

Medical Terminology - Other Prefixes	
Term	**Meaning**
dys-	difficult or without pain
mal-	bad, poor
neo-	new
syn-	together
tachy-	fast

Medical Terminology - Other Roots	
Term	**Meaning**
necr/o	dead
noct/i	night
par/o	bear
phag/o	eat
phil/o	attraction
plast/o	repair, formation
pyr/o	fire, fever
scler/o	tough, hard
sinistr/o	left
syphil/o	syphilis
therap/o	treatment
therm/o	heat
thromb/o	thrombosis
troph/o	development

Medical Terminology - Other Suffixes	
Term	**Meaning**
algia	pain
ar	pertaining to
centesis	puncture
clysis	irrigation
ectasia	dilatation, dilation
ectomy	excision
emes/is	vomiting
emia	blood
esthesia	feelings
genesis, gen/o	development, formation, beginning
gnosis	know
ia	noun ending
ia, ic	pertaining to
it is	inflammation
manual	hand
meter	measuring instrument
oid	resembling
ologist	one who studies
ology	study of
oma	tumor
opia	vision
orrhagia	hemorrhage
orrhaphy	suture

Medical Terminology - Other Suffixes	
Term	**Meaning**
orrhea	flow
orrhexis	rupture
osis	condition of
ostomy	new opening
otomy	incision
pedal	foot
pexy	fixing, fixation
phob/ia	fear
plasm	growth
plegia, plegic	paralysis
ptosis	drooping
scope, scopy	examining, looking at
spasm	twitching
sperm	sperm
stasis	slow, stop
tome	instrument
tripsy	crushing

Notes

Scoring Sheets (tear out & copy)

1) A B C D
2) A B C D
3) A B C D
4) A B C D
5) A B C D
6) A B C D
7) A B C D
8) A B C D
9) A B C D
10) A B C D
11) A B C D
12) A B C D
13) A B C D
14) A B C D
15) A B C D
16) A B C D
17) A B C D
18) A B C D
19) A B C D
20) A B C D
21) A B C D
22) A B C D
23) A B C D
24) A B C D
25) A B C D
26) A B C D
27) A B C D
28) A B C D
29) A B C D
30) A B C D
31) A B C D
32) A B C D
33) A B C D
34) A B C D
35) A B C D
36) A B C D
37) A B C D
38) A B C D
39) A B C D
40) A B C D
41) A B C D
42) A B C D
43) A B C D
44) A B C D
45) A B C D
46) A B C D
47) A B C D
48) A B C D
49) A B C D
50) A B C D
51) A B C D
52) A B C D
53) A B C D
54) A B C D
55) A B C D
56) A B C D
57) A B C D
58) A B C D
59) A B C D
60) A B C D
61) A B C D
62) A B C D
63) A B C D
64) A B C D
65) A B C D
66) A B C D
67) A B C D
68) A B C D
69) A B C D
70) A B C D
71) A B C D
72) A B C D
73) A B C D
74) A B C D
75) A B C D
76) A B C D
77) A B C D
78) A B C D
79) A B C D
80) A B C D
81) A B C D
82) A B C D
83) A B C D
84) A B C D
85) A B C D
86) A B C D
87) A B C D
88) A B C D
89) A B C D
90) A B C D
91) A B C D
92) A B C D
93) A B C D
94) A B C D
95) A B C D
96) A B C D
97) A B C D
98) A B C D
99) A B C D
100) A B C D

XXXXXXXXXXXXX
XXXXXXXXXXXXX
XXXXXXXXXXXXX
XXXXXXXXXXXXX

Scoring Sheet

(tear out & copy)

1) A B C D	31) A B C D	61) A B C D	91) A B C D
2) A B C D	32) A B C D	62) A B C D	92) A B C D
3) A B C D	33) A B C D	63) A B C D	93) A B C D
4) A B C D	34) A B C D	64) A B C D	94) A B C D
5) A B C D	35) A B C D	65) A B C D	95) A B C D
6) A B C D	36) A B C D	66) A B C D	96) A B C D
7) A B C D	37) A B C D	67) A B C D	97) A B C D
8) A B C D	38) A B C D	68) A B C D	98) A B C D
9) A B C D	39) A B C D	69) A B C D	99) A B C D
10) A B C D	40) A B C D	70) A B C D	100) A B C D
11) A B C D	41) A B C D	71) A B C D	
12) A B C D	42) A B C D	72) A B C D	XXXXXXXXXXXXX
13) A B C D	43) A B C D	73) A B C D	XXXXXXXXXXXXX
14) A B C D	44) A B C D	74) A B C D	XXXXXXXXXXXXX
15) A B C D	45) A B C D	75) A B C D	XXXXXXXXXXXXX
16) A B C D	46) A B C D	76) A B C D	
17) A B C D	47) A B C D	77) A B C D	
18) A B C D	48) A B C D	78) A B C D	
19) A B C D	49) A B C D	79) A B C D	
20) A B C D	50) A B C D	80) A B C D	
21) A B C D	51) A B C D	81) A B C D	
22) A B C D	52) A B C D	82) A B C D	
23) A B C D	53) A B C D	83) A B C D	
24) A B C D	54) A B C D	84) A B C D	
25) A B C D	55) A B C D	85) A B C D	
26) A B C D	56) A B C D	86) A B C D	
27) A B C D	57) A B C D	87) A B C D	
28) A B C D	58) A B C D	88) A B C D	
29) A B C D	59) A B C D	89) A B C D	
30) A B C D	60) A B C D	90) A B C D	

Scoring Sheet

(tear out & copy)

1) A B C D
2) A B C D
3) A B C D
4) A B C D
5) A B C D
6) A B C D
7) A B C D
8) A B C D
9) A B C D
10) A B C D
11) A B C D
12) A B C D
13) A B C D
14) A B C D
15) A B C D
16) A B C D
17) A B C D
18) A B C D
19) A B C D
20) A B C D
21) A B C D
22) A B C D
23) A B C D
24) A B C D
25) A B C D
26) A B C D
27) A B C D
28) A B C D
29) A B C D
30) A B C D
31) A B C D
32) A B C D
33) A B C D
34) A B C D
35) A B C D
36) A B C D
37) A B C D
38) A B C D
39) A B C D
40) A B C D
41) A B C D
42) A B C D
43) A B C D
44) A B C D
45) A B C D
46) A B C D
47) A B C D
48) A B C D
49) A B C D
50) A B C D
51) A B C D
52) A B C D
53) A B C D
54) A B C D
55) A B C D
56) A B C D
57) A B C D
58) A B C D
59) A B C D
60) A B C D
61) A B C D
62) A B C D
63) A B C D
64) A B C D
65) A B C D
66) A B C D
67) A B C D
68) A B C D
69) A B C D
70) A B C D
71) A B C D
72) A B C D
73) A B C D
74) A B C D
75) A B C D
76) A B C D
77) A B C D
78) A B C D
79) A B C D
80) A B C D
81) A B C D
82) A B C D
83) A B C D
84) A B C D
85) A B C D
86) A B C D
87) A B C D
88) A B C D
89) A B C D
90) A B C D
91) A B C D
92) A B C D
93) A B C D
94) A B C D
95) A B C D
96) A B C D
97) A B C D
98) A B C D
99) A B C D
100) A B C D

XXXXXXXXXXXXX
XXXXXXXXXXXXX
XXXXXXXXXXXXX
XXXXXXXXXXXXX

Scoring Sheet

(tear out & copy)

1) A B C D	31) A B C D	61) A B C D	91) A B C D
2) A B C D	32) A B C D	62) A B C D	92) A B C D
3) A B C D	33) A B C D	63) A B C D	93) A B C D
4) A B C D	34) A B C D	64) A B C D	94) A B C D
5) A B C D	35) A B C D	65) A B C D	95) A B C D
6) A B C D	36) A B C D	66) A B C D	96) A B C D
7) A B C D	37) A B C D	67) A B C D	97) A B C D
8) A B C D	38) A B C D	68) A B C D	98) A B C D
9) A B C D	39) A B C D	69) A B C D	99) A B C D
10) A B C D	40) A B C D	70) A B C D	100) A B C D
11) A B C D	41) A B C D	71) A B C D	
12) A B C D	42) A B C D	72) A B C D	XXXXXXXXXXXXX
13) A B C D	43) A B C D	73) A B C D	XXXXXXXXXXXXX
14) A B C D	44) A B C D	74) A B C D	XXXXXXXXXXXXX
15) A B C D	45) A B C D	75) A B C D	XXXXXXXXXXXXX
16) A B C D	46) A B C D	76) A B C D	
17) A B C D	47) A B C D	77) A B C D	
18) A B C D	48) A B C D	78) A B C D	
19) A B C D	49) A B C D	79) A B C D	
20) A B C D	50) A B C D	80) A B C D	
21) A B C D	51) A B C D	81) A B C D	
22) A B C D	52) A B C D	82) A B C D	
23) A B C D	53) A B C D	83) A B C D	
24) A B C D	54) A B C D	84) A B C D	
25) A B C D	55) A B C D	85) A B C D	
26) A B C D	56) A B C D	86) A B C D	
27) A B C D	57) A B C D	87) A B C D	
28) A B C D	58) A B C D	88) A B C D	
29) A B C D	59) A B C D	89) A B C D	
30) A B C D	60) A B C D	90) A B C D	

Resources

Exam Preparation Products We Recommend

Medical Coding Exam System
http://medicalcodingexamsystem.com

Faster Coder - Code Faster - Code Better
http://fastercoder.com

Other Resources

Elite Members Area – 7 day FREE trial!
http://medicalcodingpromembers.com

Medical Coding Pro – We have Exam Study Guides for almost all medical coding certifications.

http://medicalcodingpro.com

We support author Annie Lee. Check out her journals, budget planners, recipe books, and other journals on Amazon.com

https://amzn.to/3bj8A9y

If you find this information helpful please leave us a review or rating. We are a small company trying to help people get certified and we appreciate any support!

MEDICAL CODING PRO

Medical Coding Pro provides information about medical coding. We also help people in the medical coding community prepare for the medical coding certification exam.

Our mission is to help everyone we can pass the exam and gain their certification as quickly as possible.To do this we offer quality exam preparation tools such as Medical Coding Practice Exams, the Medical Coding Exam System, the Medical Coding Exam Strategy and the Medical Coding Pro Elite Members Area.

Visit us on the web at:

www.MedicalCodingPro.com

www.MedicalCodingProMembers.com

www.MedicalCodingExamSystem.com

www.MedicalCodingNews.org

Made in the USA
Las Vegas, NV
07 April 2023

70300777R00096